Periodontal re-evaluation
the scientific way

Jan Egelberg & Noel Claffey

Periodontal re-evaluation

– the scientific way

Munksgaard

Periodontal re-evaluation – the scientific way
1st edition, 1st printing

Composition and typesetting by Tegneren Jens ApS, Vejle
Printed in Denmark 1994, by Special-Trykkeriet Viborg a/s

ISBN 87-16-11375-6

Contents

Preface

The following text consists of a compilation of clinical studies on initial periodontal therapy. The purpose of the book is to present some essential information relative to the evaluation of the outcome of this therapy. The information is presented in the light of our need for scientific data to justify our therapeutic procedures.

A limited number of investigations have been reviewed. Furthermore, emphasis has been placed on studies by ourselves and our co-workers. For some aspects, a large number of studies are available and could have been reviewed. For other aspects, studies are few or are lacking, which has been a shortcoming in our efforts to present a review with a reasonable degree of comprehensiveness.

A uniform and condensed mode has been used to present the various studies. Following the presentation of procedures and results for each study, we have added some comments of our own. The research reviews are not intended to be detailed. For a deeper and more critical understanding of the various studies presented, the reader should scrutinize the original research papers. This text may best serve its purpose when the need to do so is felt.

In addition to reviews of clinical studies, we have included 2 series of case reports of patients participating in our own studies in order to further illustrate the problems encountered in re-evaluation. Towards the end of the book we give some personal views on practical aspects of periodontal re-evaluation in light of the research that has been reviewed.

This book could prove useful for periodontists, dentists and hygienists who require an update on research relating to periodontal re-evaluation. Post-doctoral students of periodontics may want to use the text as an introduction or as a background reference for their studies. This book should also be useful for undergraduate dental students interested in the scientific basis for initial periodontal therapy.

We would like to acknowledge our co-workers in this research over the years as well as all other colleagues and researchers contributing to present-day knowledge and understanding. Their work made this book possible.

June 1994
Jan Egelberg
Noel Claffey

CHAPTER 1

Introduction

Evaluation of initial periodontal treatment

Treatment of chronic periodontitis in adults is generally initiated with oral hygiene instruction followed by supra- and subgingival debridement of the teeth (scaling and root planing). This phase of the therapy is commonly termed initial periodontal treatment.

A few months after completion, the result of the initial treatment is usually evaluated to assess the need for repeated initial procedures and the need for supplementary periodontal surgery.

Re-evaluation of results following initial treatment is critical for adequate selection of additional therapy and for establishing the best possible long-term prognosis. The therapist needs to be familiar with the current state of knowledge in the following areas:

- validity and limitations of the various examination methods used to evaluate the disease process;

- degree of healing to be expected as observed from the clinical records; and

- the usefulness of the different clinical signs in predicting and evaluating the short- and long-term outcomes of treatment.

It will become obvious to the reader of this text that re-evaluation after initial periodontal treatment cannot, as yet, be performed solely on a scientific basis. In the absence of clear guidelines, it is necessary to employ subjective judgments as well. However, it is important that each clinician be aware of what is known and what is unknown from scientific studies of the various problems.

It should be added that the term *initial treatment* is not ideal, since the therapy is commonly performed with the intention of being definitive in itself. In most studies, the authors seem to have had such an intention, as is evidenced from the use of local anesthetics during treatment, a probable prerequisite for the performance of thorough subgingival debridement.

Clinical examination

Evaluation of initial periodontal treatment is commonly based on records of dental plaque, bleeding on probing, suppuration on probing and probing depth obtained at 4-6 sites around each tooth. In clinical practice, completeness of these records may vary. In scientific studies, detailed records are necessary for an adequate and objective description of the healing events.

Changes of probing attachment levels

Periodontal attachment levels are recorded by measuring the distance between the probe tip and the cementoenamel junction. A reduction of this distance after therapy as compared with before therapy is taken as a sign of improvement. Conversely, an increase in this distance indicates deterioration.

It is important to realize that the location of the probe tip during probing may not correspond to the histological connective tissue attachment level at the site. Hence, the clinical findings are termed probing attachment level measurements.

Probing attachment levels are usually not recorded in clinical practice due to the cumbersome nature of these measurements. In scientific studies, however, observations of changes in probing attachment levels are used as a method of monitoring the healing events at the base of the periodontal pocket.

The determination of changes of probing attachment levels at individual tooth sites by comparison of a single measurement after treatment to a single measurement before treatment is hampered by limitations in the reproducibility of the measurements. Investigators have attempted to compensate for this by the use of repeated recordings.

Duplicate measurements before therapy can be compared with duplicate recordings after treatment in 2 different ways, as illustrated on the following page:

- for comparison of the means of the duplicates; or

- for determination of the presence or absence of an overlap between the duplicate recordings before and after treatment (gap method).

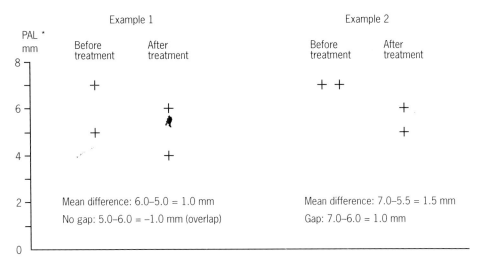

Fig. 1-1. Examples of comparisons of duplicate end-point probing attachment level measurements.
* PAL = probing attachment level = probe tip to cementoenamel junction

The mean difference is calculated by subtracting the mean of the 2 measurements after treatment from the mean of the 2 measurements before treatment.

With the gap method one looks for an absence of overlap and the magnitude of the gap between the pairs of measurements before and after treatment. For instance, to determine gain of attachment, the higher of the 2 recordings after treatment is compared with the lower of the 2 recordings before treatment.

In example 1, the mean difference of 1.0 mm could well reflect difficulties during probing and resultant measurement errors, since there is an overlap of the duplicate pairs of measurements. In example 2, it seems probable that the mean difference of 1.5 mm reflects a true change (gain of probing attachment level), since there is no overlap between the pairs of recordings. Furthermore, the gap of 1.0 mm between pre-treatment values and the higher of the post-treatment recordings reinforces the probability of a real change having occurred.

Probing attachment level change can also be assessed by subjecting a series of measurements obtained at intervals during the observation period to statistical evaluation using linear regression analysis. The following graph presents an example of such an analysis for an individual tooth site.

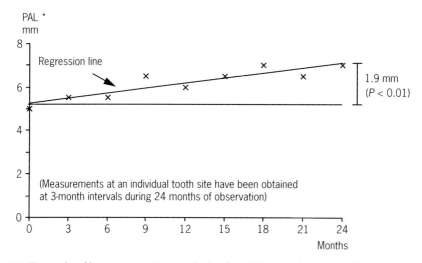

Fig. 1-2. Example of linear regression analysis of probing attachment level measurements.
* PAL = probing attachment level = probe tip to cementoenamel junction

The line of best fit (regression line) for all the measurements over time is calculated. The projected difference between the 2 end-points of this line on the
y-axis is determined (1.9 mm probing attachment loss in the example). The
analysis includes a statistical evaluation to assure that the slope of the regression line reflects a true gradual change of the data points, as opposed to
a slope formed by scattered data points due to unreliable measurements (in
the example the probability for random change is less than 1%; $P < 0.01$).

Identification of sites showing change of probing attachment level can be
made using different requirements for magnitude of change over the observation interval (threshold for change): for example, ≥ 1.0 mm, ≥ 1.5 mm etc.
Similarly, the requirement for statistical probability can be set at different
levels.

The use of regression analysis to determine changes of probing attachment
levels has certain limitations. For instance, regression analysis is more suited
to a gradual change throughout rather than to a sudden change encountered
at either the beginning or end of the observation interval. As no single
method may be ideal, investigators may combine the use of a couple of
methods for identification of sites showing probing attachment change.

CHAPTER 2

Methods of evaluation

The evaluation of periodontal tissues commonly includes examinations for the presence of dental plaque and calculus, bleeding and suppuration on probing, probing depths and radiographic evaluation. The interpretation of these records should be based on knowledge of their validity and limitations. Varying numbers of studies are available for each examination method. The studies reviewed herein address the following questions:

• What variation in probing forces can be observed among various clinicians during probing depth measurements? How painful is periodontal probing to the patients?

• What extent of connective tissue inflammation is associated with sites that bleed on probing as compared with sites that do not bleed? To what extent is bleeding on probing related to the probing force used? To what extent are bleeding scores at individual sites reproducible?

• What is the apical extent of penetration of the probe tip in relation to the base of the junctional epithelium? To what extent will the probing measurements vary following use of different probing forces? How reproducible are recordings of probing depth?

• To what extent is it feasible to evaluate the root surfaces for the presence of residual subgingival calculus in order to assess the quality of scaling and root planing?

• Is the presence or absence of a crestal lamina dura on radiographs related to the inflammatory status of the interdental gingiva?

HASSELL ET AL.[48] studied the probing force used by various clinicians during probing depth measurements.

Subjects and procedures

- 5 patients with varying degrees of periodontal involvement

- measurements on 4 aspects of mandibular right incisors, canine, premo-lars and first molar

- pressure-sensitive probe; probe tip diameter not reported

- computation of mean forces used by each of 6 experienced clinicians dur-ing probing depth measurements

Results

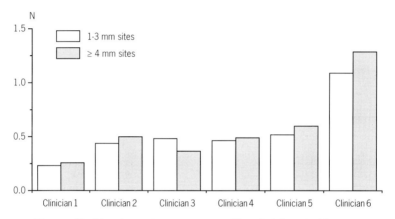

Fig. 2-1. Probing forces in newtons used by clinicians 1-6 for sites 1-3 mm and ≥ 4 mm deep

Comments

- Although the mean probing forces used by the clinicians ranged from about 0.25 N to about 1.25 N, 4 of the 6 clinicians used forces of about 0.50 N.

- Similar forces were used in sites 1-3 mm and ≥ 4 mm deep.

- Freed et al.[36] studied the probing forces used among 4 groups of clinicians (dental students, general dentists, dental hygienists and periodontists) and found a similar range of forces as those above for all groups of clini-cians. In addition, Freed et al. found that greater forces were used in pos-terior than in anterior segments of the dentition.

HEFT ET AL.[49] studied the degree of painfulness of periodontal probing to patients before and after initial periodontal treatment.

Subjects and procedures

- 46 gingivitis patients provided with initial periodontal treatment

- recordings of visual gingival inflammation, bleeding on probing and probing depth at 6 sites around all teeth at baseline, after 1 month and after 3 months

- standardized probing force: 0.25 N; probe tip diameter: 0.40 mm

- subjects asked to rate the overall pain experience after each examination by placing a crosshatch on a 150-mm line between extremes of no pain and the most pain imaginable (visual analog scale)

Results

Table 2-1
Visual inflammation, bleeding on probing and visual analog scale reading at baseline
and after 1 and 3 months

Measurement	Baseline	1 month	3 months
Visual inflammation*	87%	42%	24%
Bleeding on probing*	74%	34%	26%
Visual analog scale reading**	65 mm	52 mm	43 mm

* Means of full-mouth percentage scores.
**Distance from "no pain" end of 150-mm scale.

Comments

- The degree of pain was seemingly related to the magnitude of the clinical scores. These results may be explained by the difference in extent of sub-gingival penetration of the probe tip in inflamed versus healthy gingiva (see pages 30-39).

- Due to the study design, it cannot be excluded that the patients experienced less pain at repeated examinations because they became accustomed to the procedure and therefore less apprehensive.

GREENSTEIN ET AL.[43] studied the extent of connective tissue inflammation in biopsies of gingiva with and without bleeding on probing.

Subjects and procedures

- 24 patients scheduled for periodontal surgery after initial periodontal treatment

- a total of 45 buccal sites tested for bleeding on probing followed by biopsy

- standardized probing force: 0.25 N; probe tip diameter: 0.35 mm

- mean probing depth: 1.8 mm (range 1-3 mm)

- presence or absence of bleeding recorded within 30 s of 3 consecutive probings

- bleeding sites, $n = 24$; nonbleeding sites, $n = 21$

- biopsies evaluated histologically for the percentage area of inflammatory cell infiltrate; outer (oral) and inner (dental) aspects evaluated separately

Results

Table 2-2
Percentage of inflamed connective tissue in biopsies of gingiva with and without bleeding on probing

Location of connective tissue	With bleeding	Without bleeding
Oral aspect of buccal biopsy	9	7
Dental aspect of buccal biopsy	45	28

Comments

- Higher levels of inflammation in the connective tissue next to the tooth were recorded for bleeding as compared with nonbleeding sites.

- Although this study of shallow buccal gingival areas demonstrates a difference between bleeding and nonbleeding sites, the nonbleeding sites were found to have appreciable inflammatory cell infiltrates.

DAVENPORT ET AL.[30] also studied the extent of connective tissue inflammation in biopsies of untreated gingiva with and without bleeding on probing.

Subjects and procedures

- 12 patients with at least 1 untreated tooth scheduled for extraction due to advanced chronic periodontitis

- a total of 14 buccal or lingual sites tested for bleeding on probing followed by biopsy

- conventional probing; probe tip diameter: 0.55 mm; presence or absence of bleeding recorded within 15 s

- mean probing depth: bleeding sites ($n = 9$):   5.2 mm
  nonbleeding sites ($n = 5$):   4.5 mm

- biopsies evaluated histologically for the percentage area of inflammatory cell infiltrate in the entire biopsy coronal to the base of the junctional epithelium

Results

Table 2-3
Percentage of inflamed connective tissue in biopsies of gingiva with and without bleeding on probing

Location of connective tissue	With bleeding	Without bleeding
Entire area of biopsy	55	31

Comments

- The authors reported that 5 of the 9 bleeding sites, but none of the nonbleeding sites, showed suppuration in addition to bleeding.

- It is possible that the histological difference between bleeding and nonbleeding gingiva would have been more apparent if counts had been restricted to the dental aspect of the gingiva (compare Greenstein et al.[43], page 16).

- All bleeding sites, but none of the nonbleeding sites, showed histological ulceration of the pocket epithelium. The number of polymorphonuclear leukocytes was markedly higher in bleeding compared with nonbleeding sites (data not shown here).

PASSO ET AL.[78] studied connective tissue inflammation in biopsies of gingiva with bleeding on probing as compared with biopsies with bleeding and suppuration on probing.

Subjects and procedures

- 9 periodontitis patients requiring periodontal surgery

- a total of 56 interproximal sites tested for bleeding/suppuration on probing followed by biopsy

- conventional probing; probe tip diameter: 0.35 mm; presence or absence of bleeding/suppuration recorded within 30 s

- bleeding sites ($n = 23$): 5.2 mm average probing depth; bleeding plus suppuration sites ($n = 33$): 4.5 mm average depth

- biopsies evaluated histologically for the percentage area of inflammatory cell infiltrate in the entire biopsy coronal to the base of the junctional epithelium

Results

Table 2-4

Percentage of inflamed connective tissue in biopsies of gingiva with bleeding and bleeding plus suppuration on probing

Location of connective tissue	Bleeding	Bleeding + suppuration
Entire area of interproximal biopsy	28	42
	(2-79)*	(5-97)*

* Range from lowest to highest.

Comments

- Although the mean percentage of inflamed connective tissue was different between bleeding and bleeding plus suppuration sites, quite some variation was observed from specimen to specimen.

- According to the authors, some of the biopsies were sectioned in a buccolingual direction, others in a mesiodistal direction. The results may have been influenced by this lack of standardization of the connective tissue area under evaluation. The counts obtained may not be comparable to the counts obtained in the studies using buccal or lingual gingival biopsies (see Greenstein et al.[43] and Davenport et al.[30], pages 16-17).

HARPER & ROBINSON[47] related bleeding on probing to the extent of connective tissue inflammation in biopsies of gingiva before and after initial periodontal treatment.

Subjects and procedures

- 16 patients with advanced chronic periodontitis and ≥ 4 interproximal sites with pocket depth ≥ 6 mm

- 3 visits, spaced 1 week apart, for oral hygiene instruction and repeated root planing

- a total of 61 interproximal sites tested for bleeding on probing followed by biopsy
  - before treatment ($n = 36$)
  - 1 week after treatment ($n = 25$)

- standardized probing forces: 0.15 N for bleeding on probing and 0.25 N for probing depth; probe tip diameter not given; presence or absence of bleeding recorded within 15 s

- biopsies evaluated histologically for the percentage area of inflammatory cell infiltrate in the entire biopsy coronal to the base of the junctional epithelium

Results

Table 2-5
Mean results before and after initial periodontal treatment

	Before treatment	After treatment
Probing depth (mm)	7.2	5.9
% bleeding sites	80	10
% inflamed connective tissue	57	30

Comments

- Overall, treatment resulted in reduced bleeding as well as reduced connective tissue inflammation. On a site level, however, the authors observed a limited association between bleeding on probing and the percentage of inflamed connective tissue (coefficients of correlation: before treatment = 0.1; after treatment = 0.3).

LANG ET AL.[60] studied the effect of different probing forces on bleeding on probing scores in subjects with healthy gingiva.

Subjects and procedures

- 12 dental hygiene students, 20-27 years of age

- subjects selected on the basis of good oral hygiene standards, clinically healthy gingival tissues and absence of probing depths > 3 mm

- daily supervised oral hygiene, starting 3 weeks pre-experimentally and continuing throughout the study

- bleeding on probing scores obtained at 2 time points, 10 days apart

- 4 sites per tooth; 28 sites from the 7 teeth in each quadrant

- the 4 quadrants in each subject randomly assigned to probing forces of 0.25 N, 0.50 N, 0.75 N and 1.00 N

- probe tip diameter: 0.40 mm

- the percentage of bleeding sites calculated for each probing force (average of the 2 time points)

Results

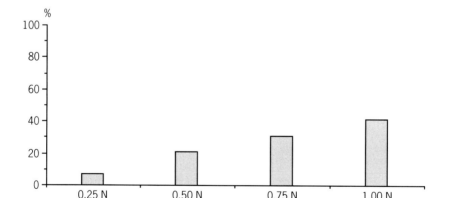

Fig. 2-2. Percentage of sites with bleeding on probing following the use of different probing forces

Comments

- The use of increasing probing forces resulted in higher bleeding scores.

- In these subjects, presumably with quite healthy gingiva, minimal bleeding was found using a probing force of 0.25 N. Therefore, this force may be most suited to discriminate between healthy and inflamed gingival tissues.

- Bleeding provoked by forces higher than 0.25 N may be caused by trauma to healthy blood vessels rather than rupture of fragile vessels in inflamed tissues.

- This study was repeated by the same investigators and the results confirmed in a group of patients with a history of successfully treated periodontal disease, that is, in patients with a reduced but healthy periodontium (Karayiannis et al.[57]).

- If probing forces above 0.25 N are preferred, one will have to accept that bleeding scores of clinically healthy gingiva may not approach 0%.

VAN DER VELDEN[90] studied the effect of different probing forces on bleeding and probing scores before and after initial periodontal treatment.

Subjects and procedures

- 6 periodontitis patients

- a total of 92 approximal sites

- oral hygiene instruction, scaling and root planing scheduled during a period of 5-10 weeks

- 4 consecutive measurements in each subject using probing forces of 0.15 N, 0.25 N, 0.50 N and 0.75 N

- probe tip diameter: 0.65 mm

- final recordings 4-5 weeks after completion of treatment

Results

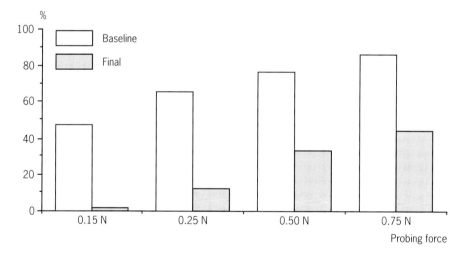

Fig. 2-3. Bleeding scores before and after treatment following the use of different probing forces

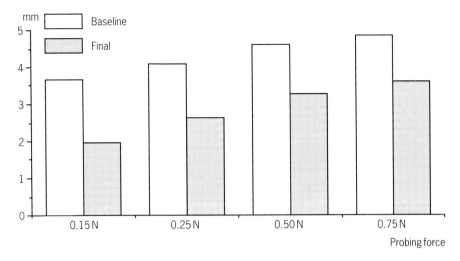

Fig. 2-4. Probing depth before and after treatment following the use of different probing forces

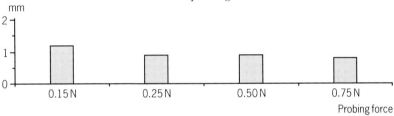

Fig. 2-5. Changes of probing attachment levels before and after treatment following the use of different probing forces

Comments

- The bleeding scores and probing depths increased with increasing probing force used.

- The difference in probing depth between the lowest and highest probing force amounted to 1-1.5 mm.

- The reductions of bleeding and probing scores, relative to baseline scores, were greatest for the lowest probing force.

- It can be argued that the increase in bleeding and probing depth scores seen with increasing probing force may to some extent be related to the repeated probings of sites rather than to the increase in probing force. However, to prepare for this study, van der Velden investigated the effect of 4 consecutive probings and found little or no increase in bleeding tendency due to the repeated probing. See also the results of Janssen et al.[52,54] on bleeding scores after repeated probings (pages 28-29). Results of other studies indicate that a second probing is only slightly affected by the first recording; on the average 0.1 mm deeper (Claffey et al.[27], Janssen et al.[55]).

CATON ET AL.[21] and PROYE ET AL.[81] also studied the effect of different probing forces on bleeding and probing scores before and after initial periodontal treatment.

Subjects and procedures

- 10 patients with ≥ 6 approximal periodontal pockets 3-7 mm deep as recorded by manual probing

- a total of 128 approximal sites

- oral hygiene instruction at baseline, reinforced at intervals during the observation period

- a single episode of scaling and root planing at baseline

- 3 consecutive measurements using probing forces of 0.15 N, 0.25 N and 0.50 N followed by "manual" probing using a conventional periodontal probe

- probe tip diameter: 0.35 mm

- 16 weeks of observation

Results

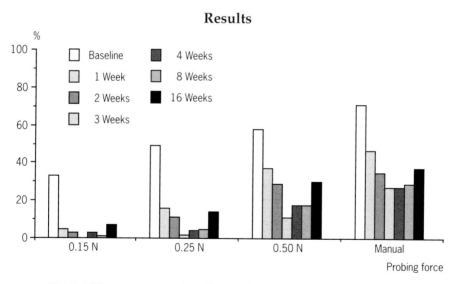

Fig. 2-6. Bleeding scores at baseline and at various intervals following treatment using different probing forces

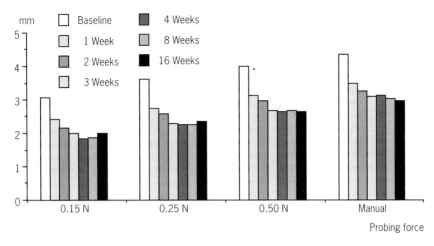

Fig. 2-7. Probing depths at baseline and at various intervals following treatment using different probing forces

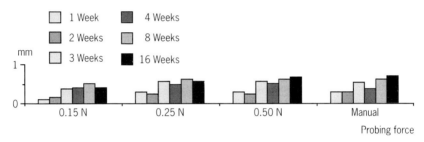

Fig. 2-8. Changes of probing attachment level at baseline and at various intervals following treatment using different probing forces

Comments

- The bleeding scores and probing depths increased with the use of increasing probing force. The highest scores were obtained following manual probing.

- The improvement in bleeding scores following treatment and the rebound tendency towards the end of the observation interval were observed for all probing forces.

- The difference in probing depth between the lowest probing force and manual probing amounted to 1-1.5 mm.

- The reductions of bleeding and probing scores, relative to their baseline values, were greater for the lower than for the higher probing forces, results similar to those of van der Velden[90] (see pages 22-23).

- Consecutive probings of sites with increasing probing forces were performed in this study, as in the study by van der Velden[90]. This needs to be considered in the interpretation of the results (see page 23).

CHAMBERLAIN ET AL.[23] evaluated the effect of nonsurgical and surgical treatment of intraosseous periodontal defects using different probing forces.

Subjects and procedures

- 14 patients with a total of 50 periodontal lesions associated with approximal intraosseous defects

- 25 lesions treated with root planing and 25 lesions treated with periodontal flap surgery

- measurements of probing depths preoperatively (2 months after initial therapy) and 6 months postoperatively

- 3 consecutive measurements using increasing probing forces: 0.25 N, 0.50 N and 0.75 N

- probe tip diameter: 0.50 mm

Results

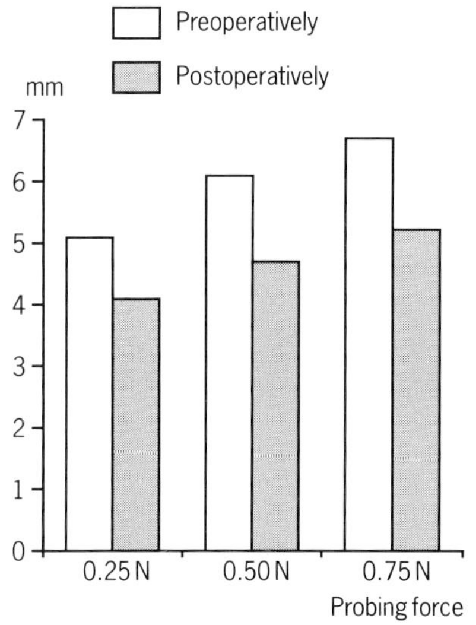

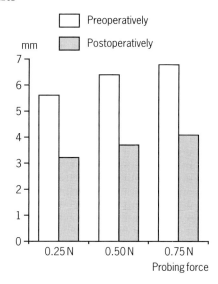

Fig. 2-9. Pre- and postoperative probing depths for nonsurgical treatment following different probing forces

Fig. 2-10. Pre- and postoperative probing depths for surgical treatment following different probing forces

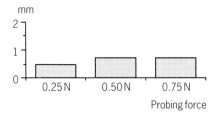

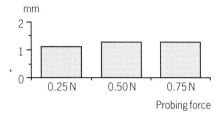

Fig. 2-11. Changes of probing attachment level for nonsurgical treatment following different probing forces

Fig. 2-12. Changes of probing attachment level for surgical treatment following different probing forces

Comments

- Probing depths increased with the use of increasing probing force.

- Similar changes in probing depth and probing attachment level following treatment could be observed for all 3 probing forces.

- The consecutive probings of the sites with increasing probing forces may to some extent have affected the probing depth results (see page 23).

- This study, and the studies of van der Velden[90], Caton et al.[21] and Proye et al.[81] (see pages 22-25) do not relate the amount of probe penetration to histological landmarks. Therefore, these studies alone should not be used to select a suitable probing force for comparison of healing events from before and after therapy (see studies on probe penetration, pages 30-39).

JANSSEN ET AL.[52,54] studied the reproducibility of bleeding on probing.

Subjects and procedures

- 13 patients, 20-60 years of age, having received initial periodontal therapy

- a total of 717 approximal sites

- mean approximal probing depth: 4.7 mm

- duplicate recordings of bleeding on probing with an interval of 100 min

- standardized probing force: 0.32 N; probe tip diameter: 0.40 mm

- probing by "searching" the site a few times

- calculation of agreement/disagreement of bleeding and nonbleeding sites between the 2 recordings

Results

Table 2-6
Number of sites with bleeding and no bleeding at the first and second examination

		Second examination		
		bleeding	**no bleeding**	
First examination	bleeding	174	91	265
	no bleeding	104	348	452
		278	439	717

Specific agreement = $174 \div \dfrac{265 + 278}{2} \times 100 = 64\%$.

Kappa = 0.42.
(Kappa statistics take into account all the numbers in a 2 × 2 table as well as chance occurrence and provide values from 0 to 1.0. Less than 0.40 represents poor agreement beyond chance, 0.40 - 0.75 fair to good agreement and 0.75 and above excellent agreement.)

Table 2-7
Number of sites with bleeding and no bleeding at first and second examination by probing depth

Probing depth (mm)	% bleeding sites		Specific agreement (%)	Kappa
	Examination 1	Examination 2		
2-3	15	16	35	0.23
4	26	35	51	0.30
5	49	54	67	0.31
6	70	65	72	0.13
7	64	67	75	0.27
8	68	66	73	0.45
9-10	57	57	72	0.35
Total	37	39	64	0.42

Comments

- The analysis of all sites showed that 265 sites (37%) bled on probing at the first examination and 278 (38%) at the second examination. Thus, the first probing did not seem to affect the overall bleeding score at the second examination.

- The results of the kappa statistics disclose a limited reproducibility of the bleeding scores.

- For clinical purposes, the results suggest that bleeding on probing may not be reliable on an individual site basis and should be interpreted with caution.

- Despite the above limitations, changes of bleeding scores for pooled sites in a patient seem to be a good indicator of overall improvement in gingival conditions as a result of treatment (see van der Velden[90], pages 22-23; Caton et al.[21] and Proye et al.[81], pages 24-25; also see Chapters 5 and 6: Case reports, pages 129-197).

FOWLER ET AL.[35] used gingival biopsies to study the position of the probe tip in relation to the apical termination of the junctional epithelium in untreated and treated periodontal lesions.

Subjects and procedures

- periodontal pockets, ≥ 6 mm deep, located on buccal surfaces of single-rooted teeth, condemned for extraction

- 12 untreated teeth from 6 subjects

- 15 treated teeth from 10 subjects

- treatment group: oral hygiene instruction; root planing in 1 visit; monitoring every second week until 3 consecutive recordings of bleeding on probing and probing depth indicated stabilization and no further improvement (the time required ranged from 10-23 weeks)

- recordings of bleeding on probing, probing depth and probing attachment level

- standardized probing force: 0.50 N; probe tip diameter: 0.40 mm

- biopsies of untreated and treated teeth including marginal buccal periodontal tissues with the probe tip in place and luted to the tooth

- histological analyses:
    - the location of the probe tip in relation to the apical termination of the junctional epithelium (most coronal connective tissue fibers inserting into the root)
    - the amount of chronic inflammatory cells in the connective tissue next to the probe tip (index count)

Results

Table 2-8
Clinical and histological measurements of untreated and treated sites

	Untreated (n = 12)	Treated (n = 15)	
		preoperative	postoperative
Clinical measurements			
Bleeding on probing (no. of sites)	12	13	1
Probing depth (mm)	6.1*	6.5	4.3
	(6.0 – 7.0)**	(6.0 – 8.5)	(3.0 – 5.5)
Reduction of probing depth (mm)			2.2
			(1.0 – 4.0)
Gingival recession (mm)			0.8
			(0.0 – 1.0)
Gain of probing attachment (mm)			1.4
			(0.0 – 3.0)
Histological measurements			
Probe tip to base of junctional epithelium (mm)	−0.5***		+0.7***
	(−1.3 – +0.1)		(−0.4 – +2.7)
Connective tissue inflammatory cell index	67		34
	(52 – 93)		(5 – 69)

*   Mean.
**   Range from lowest to highest.
***   + = coronal to the base, − = apical to the base.

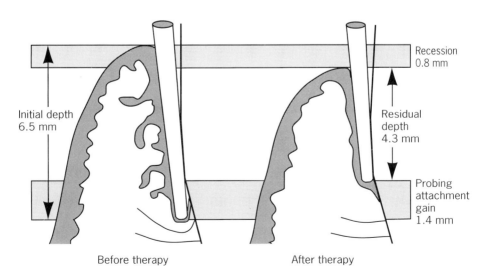

Initial depth 6.5 mm

Recession 0.8 mm

Residual depth 4.3 mm

Probing attachment gain 1.4 mm

Before therapy   After therapy

Fig. 2-13. Schematic illustration of results

Comments

- In untreated buccal sites, the probe tip generally penetrated slightly apical to the base of the junctional epithelium using a probing force of 0.50 N and a probe tip diameter of 0.40 mm.

- In the majority of the treated buccal sites, the probe tip stopped coronal to the base of the junctional epithelium.

- The difference in probe penetration between untreated and treated sites was 1.2 mm. This difference approximates the 1.4-mm gain of probing attachment level seen in the clinical findings for the treated sites.

- The connective tissue inflammatory cell index was substantially lower in the treated than the untreated specimens. However, treated specimens continued to show chronic inflammatory cells in spite of the marked clinical evidence of healing. This concurs with the results of Greenstein et al.[43] (see page 16) and Harper & Robinson[47] (see page 19).

- The schematic drawing on the previous page, based on the results for the treated sites, uses a position for the probe tip that was extrapolated from the biopsy results of untreated sites.

- In the schematic drawing, the left portion (before treatment) and the right portion (after treatment) have been lined up as if there was no change in the level of connective tissue attachment due to treatment. Although there seems to be no evidence in the literature that root planing results in improved connective tissue attachment levels, the possibility of apical displacement of the attachment level due to trauma from instrumentation needs to be considered (see Claffey et al.[27] and Claffey[25], pages 81-85).

SPRAY ET AL.[88], GARNICK ET AL.[37], POLSON ET AL.[80] and CATON ET AL.[20] also used gingival biopsies to study the position of the probe tip in relation to the apical termination of the junctional epithelium during probing of periodontal lesions.

Overview of results

Table 2-9
Probe penetration and experimental conditions

Author	Subjects, teeth and sites	Gingival status/ bleeding on probing	Tip diameter (mm) Force (N)	Probing depth (mm)	Probe tip penetration (mm)
Polson et al.[80]	19 buccal sites in teeth scheduled for surgery after initial treatment (11 patients)	No visual signs of gingivitis	0.35 mm 0.25 N	1.7 (1 – 3)**	+ 0.3*
Caton et al.[20]	45 buccal sites in teeth scheduled for surgery (24 patients)	Without visual gingivitis (n = 28)	0.35 mm 0.25 N	1.8 (1 – 3)	+ 0.2
		With visual gingivitis (n = 17)			0.0
	Same material as above	Nonbleeding (n = 21)			+ 0.2
		Bleeding (n = 24)			+ 0.1
Spray et al.[88]	8 buccal sites in untreated teeth condemned for extraction (8 patients)	Visual signs of gingivitis	0.40 mm 0.15- 0.20 N	***	– 0.1 (–1.0 – + 0.2)
Garnick et al.[37]	7 buccal sites in untreated teeth condemned for extraction (7 patients)	Bleeding on probing + visual gingivitis	0.35 mm 0.15- 0.20 N	4-8	– 0.1 (– 0.6 – + 0.5)

*   Probe tip to base of junctional epithelium; + = coronal to, – = apical to base.
**   Range from lowest to highest.
*** Not reported.

Comments

- In shallow buccal sites, without clinical signs of inflammation, Polson et al.[80] and Caton et al.[20] found that the probe tip, on average, stopped 0.2-0.3 mm short of the apical termination of the junctional epithelium using a probing force of 0.25 N and a probe tip diameter of 0.35. In the presence of visual signs of gingival inflammation, the probe tip reached the apical end of the junctional epithelium.

- In inflamed buccal sites, Spray et al.[88] and Garnick et al.[37] observed that the probe tip, on average, penetrated slightly beyond the base of the junctional epithelium using a probing force of 0.15-0.20 N and a probe tip diameter of 0.40.

ROBINSON & VITEK[83] compared clinical measurements of probe penetration to the most coronal connective tissue attachment determined after extraction of the teeth.

Subjects and procedures

- 51 incisors and premolars designated for extraction due to orthodontic, prosthetic or periodontal reasons

- a total of 131 sites

- degree of gingival inflammation at the sites scored 0, 1, 2 or 3

- probing force either 0.20 N, 0.25 N or 0.30 N; probe tip diameter: 0.35 mm

- clinical probe penetration recorded from a reference groove on the crown of the tooth

- subsequent to extraction, measurement of the distance from the reference groove to the coronal level of the periodontal ligament

- comparison of the 2 measurements for subgroups of sites with various probing forces and gingivitis scores

Results

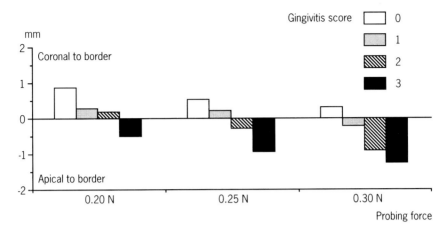

Fig. 2-14. Probe penetration in relation to coronal border of connective tissue attachment by probing force and gingivitis score

Comments

- The mean probe penetration increased with increasing probing force and with increasing gingival inflammation.

VAN DER VELDEN[89,91] and SIMONS & WATTS[87] also related clinical measurements of probe penetration to the most coronal connective tissue attachment determined after extraction of the teeth.

Overview of results

Table 2-10
Probe penetration and experimental conditions

Author	Subjects, teeth and sites	Gingival status/ bleeding on probing	Tip diameter (mm) Force (N)	Probing depth (mm)	Probe tip penetration (mm)
van der Velden[89]	58 approximal sites in 21 molars condemned for extraction after initial periodontal treatment (13 patients)	Bleeding for 45% of all sites	0.65 mm 0.50 N 0.75 N 1.00 N 1.25 N	4.0 4.4 5.0 5.2	+ 0.3* 0.0 − 0.7 − 0.8
van der Velden[91]	Same material as above	Nonbleeding (n = 32)	0.65 mm 0.75 N	4.4	+ 0.1 **(−1 − +1)
		Bleeding (n = 26)			− 0.3 (−2 − +1)
Simons & Watts[87]	60 sites around 11 un-treated teeth requiring extraction due to peri-odontal disease (4 patients)	Inflamed (n = 26)	0.65 mm 0.25 N	2.3	+ 0.9
		Inflamed (n = 34)		5.6	+ 1.5

* Probe tip to base of junctional epithelium; + = coronal to, − = apical to base.
** Range from lowest to highest.

Comments

- Compared with the other studies on probe penetration, van der Velden[89,91] used a larger probe tip diameter and greater probing forces. Nevertheless, van der Velden's results also indicate that probe penetration varies with the probing force used and the degree of gingival inflammation.

- Simons & Watts[87] also used a larger probe tip diameter but combined with a low probing force. This resulted in limited probe penetration, particularly noteworthy for the deeper untreated pockets. These authors reported a range of probe penetration varying from 2 mm apical to 6 mm coronal to the connective tissue border.

- The results of the above studies suggest that a probe tip of 0.65 mm diameter should be combined with a probing force approximating 0.75 N to reach the coronal connective tissue in the average untreated pocket. However, there seems to be quite some variation in depth of penetration from site to site.

ISIDOR ET AL.[50] studied intraexaminer reproducibility of probing depth measurements before and after periodontal treatment.

Subjects and procedures

- 17 patients with advanced periodontitis

- measurements from nonmolar teeth only; 6 sites per tooth

- duplicate measurements, 3 weeks apart, by 1 examiner both prior to and 3 months after completion of periodontal treatment

- probing "using gentle pressure" (nonstandardized probing force); probe tip diameter: 0.40 mm

- probe with 2-mm increments; readings to the nearest 1 mm

Results

Table 2-11
Percentage of sites with various magnitudes of difference between duplicate probing depth measurements before and after treatment

Difference between duplicate recordings	Before treatment	After treatment
0 mm	60	66
± 1 mm	35	30
± 2 mm	4	4
± 3 mm	1	0

Comments

- About 95% of the recordings were duplicated within 1 mm deviation. About 5% showed a difference of 2-3 mm.

- The reproducibility was somewhat improved following treatment. This is most likely related to the reduced probing depth after therapy (see Badersten et al.[6], pages 42-43; Loos et al.[65], page 44).

BADERSTEN ET AL.[6] studied both intra- and interexaminer reproducibility of probing depth measurements.

Subjects and procedures

- 16 patients with advanced periodontitis

- probing depths 1-12 mm

- measurements from nonmolar teeth only; 6 sites per tooth

- duplicate measurements, 1 week apart, by each of 2 examiners

- nonstandardized probing force; probe tip diameter: 0.50 mm

- probe with 1-mm increments; reading to the nearest 0.5 mm

Results

Table 2-12

Percentage of sites with various magnitudes of difference between duplicate probing depth measurements for intra- and interexaminer comparisons

Difference between duplicate recordings	Intraexaminer		Interexaminer	
	Examiner 1 0/1 week	Examiner 2 0/1 week	Examiner 1/2 0 week	Examiner 1/2 1 week
0 mm	33	38	35	38
± 0.5 mm	35	29	37	36
± 1.0 mm	20	21	18	17
± 1.5 mm	6	5	4	4
± 2.0 mm	3	4	3	3
± ≥ 2.5 mm	3	3	3	2

Comments

- The findings of this study are similar to those of Isidor et al.[50], also examining nonmolar teeth only (see pages 40-41).

- A comparison to the results of Isidor et al.[50], taking readings to the nearest 1 mm, suggests that readings to the nearest 0.5 mm do not seem to offer any advantage.

- Experienced and previously calibrated examiners were used, which may explain the similarity of intraexaminer and interexaminer findings.

- In addition, Badersten et al. found that (data not shown here):
  - Recordings from shallower sites were more reproducible than those from deeper sites.
  - Recordings from buccal sites were more reproducible than those from approximal sites.
  - Recordings from incisors were more reproducible than those from cuspids and premolars.
  - Recordings after treatment were more reproducible than those before treatment.
  - Reproducibility varied among patients.

These results suggest that probing depth, access and visibility are factors of importance for reproducibility of probing measurements.

LOOS ET AL.[65] studied interexaminer reproducibility of probing attachment level measurements for sites of different probing depth and location.

Subjects and procedures

- 16 patients with moderate to severe periodontitis; probing depth ranging from 0.5-9.5 mm

- recordings from 6 sites in nonmolar teeth, 8 sites in maxillary molars and 10 sites in mandibular molars (in order to include furcation sites and buccal/lingual sites of all roots, see page 130)

- margins of onlays used as reference points for the probing attachment level measurements

- duplicate measurements at the same visit by 2 examiners

- standardized probing force: 0.50 N; probe tip diameter: 0.40 mm; 1-mm increments; readings to the nearest 0.5 mm

Results

Table 2-13

Percentage of sites with various magnitudes of difference between duplicate probing attachment level measurements by probing depth and site location

Difference between dupli-cate recordings	Probing depth (mm)			Site location		
	≤ 3.5	4.0-6-5	≥ 7.0	Nonmolar sites	Molar flat surfaces*	Molar furcations
0 mm	40	32	29	36	30	33
± 0.5 mm	38	41	30	40	35	30
± 1.0 mm	15	16	19	15	16	23
± 1.5 mm	4	6	10	6	7	6
± 2.0 mm	1	2	6	1	5	3
± ≥ 2.5 mm	2	3	5	2	7	6

* Molar sites other than those at the location of the furcation apertures.

Comments

- Deviations of duplicate probings amounting to ≥ 2 mm occurred in 3% of sites ≤ 3.5 mm deep as compared with 11% of sites ≥ 7 mm deep, and in 3% of nonmolar sites as compared with 9-12% of molar sites.

SIMONS & WATTS[87] studied intraexaminer reproducibility of probing depth measurements with and without the use of standardized probing force.

Subjects and procedures

- 14 patients with moderate to severe periodontitis

- measurements from the entire dentition; 6 sites per tooth

- duplicate measurements, 1 week apart, by 1 examiner
  - standardized probing: probing force 0.25 N
  - nonstandardized probing

- Probe tip diameter: 0.64 mm; 2-mm increments; readings to the nearest 1 mm

Results

Table 2-14
Percentage sites with various magnitudes of difference between duplicate probing depth measurements for standardized and nonstandardized probing force

Difference between duplicate recordings	Standardized probing force	Nonstandardized probing force
0 mm	57	57
± 1 mm	30	31
± 2 mm	10	9
± 3 mm	3	3

Comments

- No difference in reproducibility was observed between the use of standardized and nonstandardized probing force.

- The reproducibility in this study was somewhat less than that of Loos et al.[65] (compare page 44).

- van der Velden & de Vries[92] and Badersten et al.[6] also compared the reproducibility of measurements with and without the use of standardized probing force and also did not observe any differences in results.

SHERMAN ET AL.[85,86] evaluated the ability of clinicians to detect residual calculus following subgingival scaling and root planing. They compared clinical and microscopic methods of calculus detection and related the calculus detection to subsequent gingival healing.

Subjects and procedures

- 7 subjects, 35-74 years of age, with chronic periodontitis

- 101 teeth condemned for extraction and available for study

- number of sites examined clinically:

nonmolar	498
molar	148
total	646

- oral hygiene instruction, reinforced at monthly intervals

- subgingival scaling and root planing at baseline using a combination of ultrasonic and hand instruments under local anesthesia

- repeated instrumentation after 1 week

- clinical determination of presence or absence of subgingival calculus by 3 independent, experienced periodontists:
  - prior to instrumentation
  - immediately after instrumentation
  - after 3 months

- clinical recordings at 0, 1, 2 and 3 months

- all teeth extracted at 3 months followed by analysis for residual calculus under × 10 magnification (461 tooth surfaces available)

- analysis of results:
  - interexaminer reproducibility of clinical calculus recordings comparing the 3 examiners
  - presence of residual calculus determined microscopically after tooth extraction
  - relationship between clinical and microscopic detection of calculus
  - gingival healing response during the 3-month observation period
  - gingival healing response in relation to clinical and microscopic presence of calculus at 3 months

Results
Interexaminer reproducibility of clinical calculus recordings comparing the 3 examiners (examples of results)

Table 2-15

Number of surfaces with and without subgingival calculus prior to instrumentation:
examiner A versus examiner B

		Examiner B		
		calculus	**no calculus**	
Examiner A	calculus	511	31	542
	no calculus	66	38	104
		577	69	646

Specific agreement for calculus detection = $511 \div \dfrac{542 + 577}{2} \times 100 = 91\%$.
Kappa = 0.36.

Table 2-16

Number of surfaces with and without subgingival calculus immediately after instrumentation:
examiner A versus examiner C

		Examiner C		
		calculus	**no calculus**	
Examiner A	calculus	40	54	94
	no calculus	116	436	552
		156	490	646

Specific agreement for calculus detection = $40 \div \dfrac{94 + 156}{2} \times 100 = 32\%$.
Kappa = 0.17.

Table 2-17

Number of surfaces with and without subgingival calculus 3 months after instrumentation:
examiner B versus examiner C

		Examiner C		
		calculus	**no calculus**	
Examiner B	calculus	64	164	228
	no calculus	59	359	418
		123	523	646

Specific agreement for calculus detection = $64 \div \dfrac{228 + 123}{2} \times 100 = 36\%$.
Kappa = 0.16

Presence of residual calculus determined microscopically after tooth extraction

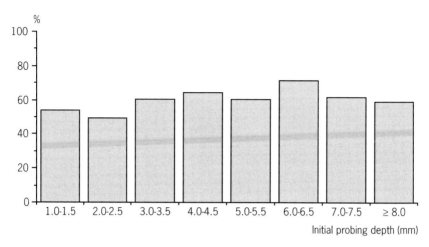

Fig. 2-15. Percentage of surfaces with residual calculus by groups of initial probing depth: microscopic detection

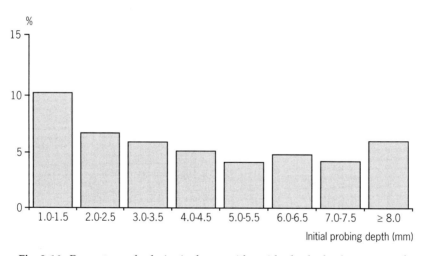

Fig. 2-16. Percentage of subgingival area with residual calculus by groups of initial probing depth: microscopic detection

Relationship between clinical and microscopic detection of calculus

Table 2-18

Number of surfaces with and without subgingival calculus: microscopic versus clinical detection 3 months after instrumentation

		Clinical detection*		
		calculus	no calculus	
Microscopic detection	calculus	60	206	266
	no calculus	23	172	195
		83	378	461

Specific agreement $= 60 \div \dfrac{266 + 83}{2} \times 100 = 34\%$.

Kappa = 0.10.
* Positive score for calculus when at least 2 of the 3 examiners had recorded the presence of calculus.

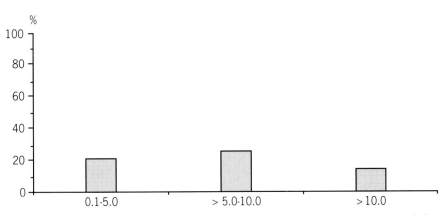

Percentage of subgingival area with residual microscopic calculus

Fig. 2-17. Percentage of surfaces with clinically detected subgingival calculus for surfaces with various amounts of microscopically observed calculus. Positive score for calculus when at least 2 of the 3 examiners had recorded calculus at 3 months

Gingival healing response during the 3-month observation period

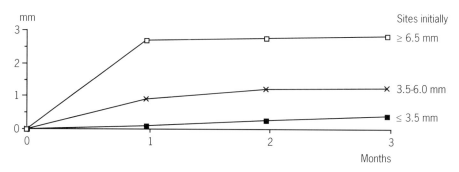

Fig. 2-18. Reduction of probing depth for sites of different initial probing depth

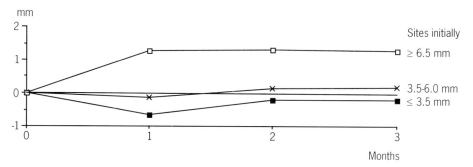

Fig. 2-19. Change of probing attachment level for sites of different initial probing depth

Gingival healing response in relation to clinical and microscopic presence of calculus at 3 months

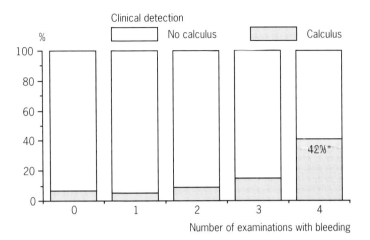

Fig. 2-20. Percentage of surfaces with and without clinical calculus at 3 months for surfaces with bleeding at 0, 1, 2, 3 or 4 examinations. Positive score for calculus when at least 2 of the 3 examiners had recorded it. *Interpretation: 42% of surfaces that showed bleeding at all 4 examinations (0, 1, 2 and 3 months) showed clinical calculus at 3 months

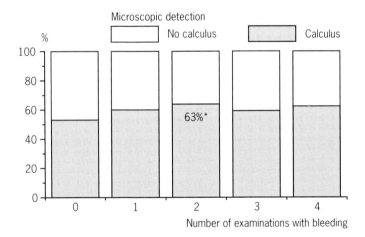

Fig. 2-21. Percentage of surfaces with and without microscopic calculus for surfaces with bleeding at 0, 1, 2, 3 or 4 examinations. * Interpretation: 63% of surfaces that showed bleeding at 2 of the 4 examinations (0, 1, 2 and 3 months) showed microscopic calculus at 3 months

Comments

- The agreement between the examiners in detecting calculus after instrumentation was low (data from only some of the comparisons presented here). This confirms findings by Biller & Kerber[14] and Pippin & Feil[79].

- Microscopically, 57% of the surfaces showed some residual calculus. On average, 5% of the subgingival surface area had remaining calculus (range 0-32%).

- The presence of residual microscopic calculus was not related to the initial probing depth at the instrumented surface. Such a relationship has been observed in other studies (Rabbani et al.[82], Caffesse et al.[19], Buchanan & Robertson[17]).

- The agreement between clinical and microscopic detection of residual calculus was low, even though the analyses had been safeguarded by use of calculus detected by at least 2 of the 3 examiners. Apparently, calculus left behind following thorough instrumentation is difficult to detect clinically.

- The changes of probing depths and probing attachment levels corresponded to those observed in other studies following initial periodontal therapy (see Badersten[3] and Badersten et al.[4,5,7,8,10], pages 60-61; Claffey et al.[29], pages 70-71; and Claffey et al.[27] and Claffey[25], pages 81-85).

- The degree of gingival healing, as evaluated from the cumulative frequency of bleeding during the study, showed some relationship to the presence of residual calculus determined clinically, but not to calculus observed microscopically. However, it can be argued that the clinical appearance of the sites may have influenced the calculus scoring.

- The authors estimate that the average surface area with residual microscopic calculus (5%) almost represents a 10-fold reduction compared with untreated control surfaces (35-40%, data not shown here). It is possible that this degree of effectiveness during root planing, leaving primarily small spots of burnished calculus behind, is sufficient for substantial gingival improvement in most situations.

- The results of this study suggest that the effectiveness of thorough subgingival debridement is best evaluated from examination of the gingival conditions a few months after instrumentation.

GREENSTEIN ET AL.[42] examined the relationship between the presence of a crestal lamina dura on radiographs and the clinical status of interdental areas.

Subjects and procedures

- 90 subjects, 21-45 years of age

- full-mouth periapical and posterior bite-wing radiographs using a long-cone technique

- each interdental area examined for presence or absence of an intact crestal lamina dura: "a consistent, radiopaque white line without any break in continuity of the superior and inferior margins"

- separate assessments from periapical and bite-wing radiographs

- clinical status of interdental areas evaluated with 4 methods:
  - visual inflammation (inflamed versus noninflamed)
  - bleeding on probing
  - presence of probing depths ≥ 4 mm
  - presence of probing attachment loss ≥ 1 mm

- if the parameter under evaluation was positive for any of the 4 locations recorded for each interdental area, the entire interdental area was scored as positive for that particular parameter

- analysis:
  - comparison of periapical and bite-wing radiographs for identification of an intact lamina dura (posterior areas only)
  - presence or absence of lamina dura, as determined from periapical radiographs, related to clinical status (entire dentition)
  - presence or absence of lamina dura, as determined from bite-wing radiographs, related to clinical status (posterior areas only)

Results

Table 2-19
Number of interdental areas with and without lamina dura:
bite-wing versus periapical radiographs

		Periapical		
		with	without	
Bite-wing	with	31	87	118
	without	111	833	944
		142	920	1062

Specific agreement $= 31 \div \dfrac{118 + 142}{2} \times 100 = 24\%$.

Kappa $= 0.13$.

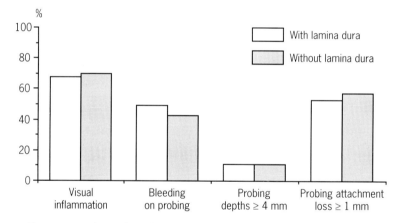

Fig. 2-22. Percentage of interdental areas with positive score (≥ 1 of 4 examined sites per interdental area) for various clinical parameters for areas with and without lamina dura (periapical radiographs)

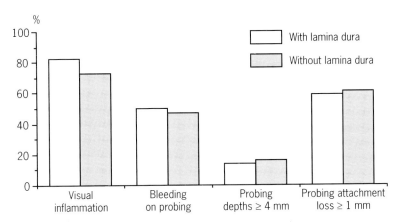

Fig. 2-23. Percentage of interdental areas with positive score (≥ 1 of 4 examined sites per interdental area) for various clinical parameters for areas with and without lamina dura (bite-wing radiographs)

Comments

- The degree of agreement for the determination of an intact lamina dura from periapical versus bite-wing radiographs was low. This may indicate that variations in X-ray projection significantly influence the radiographic image of the interdental bone crest. This, in turn, would seem to infer that the use of presence or absence of lamina dura as a diagnostic sign for interdental inflammation is questionable.

- Similar numbers of interdental areas exhibited clinical signs of inflammation irrespective of the presence or absence of lamina dura. This was observed for both periapical and bite-wing radiographs. This finding adds further doubt as to the value of an intact lamina dura as a diagnostic sign.

- Analyses of the results using increased requirements for positive clinical scores might have been of interest: for example, a positive score would have required visual inflammation plus bleeding on probing plus probing depth ≥ 4 mm for at least 2 of the 4 locations.

(The use of conventional radiographic techniques to evaluate the results of treatment is discussed in Chapter 3: Effect of initial periodontal treatment, pages 90-94.)

GENERAL COMMENTS

- What is a suitable probe tip diameter and what force should be used during periodontal probing? A primary concern in answering this question is the degree of comfort to the patient during examination. The findings of Heft et al.[49] indicate that patients perceive probing as more painful prior to initial periodontal treatment than after treatment. Since there appears to be no study specifically addressing what probing force the majority of patients find acceptable, we will have to assume that probing forces up to 0.50 N, in combination with a probe tip diameter of 0.35-0.50 mm, are tolerable to most individuals, simply because they have often been used in the available studies on periodontal probing.

- For the purpose of recording bleeding on probing, a low probing force that creates limited unwarranted traumatization seems preferable, such as 0.25 N. This force, in combination with a probe tip diameter of 0.35-0.40 mm, also seems to provide satisfactory penetration relative to the periodontal attachment level. In addition, this force/diameter combination appears adequate for overall evaluation of the outcome of periodontal treatment with respect to changes in bleeding scores, probing depths and probing attachment levels.

- van der Velden[89,91] has found that a probe tip diameter of 0.65 mm in combination with a probing force of 0.50-0.75 N provides a desirable average probe penetration relative to the periodontal attachment level. Also, van der Velden[90] has observed that this force and diameter combination is adequate for overall evaluation of the effect of treatment using bleeding scores, probing depths and probing attachment levels. However, the findings of van der Velden[89] and Simons & Watts[87] indicate that a probe tip of diameter 0.65 mm combined with a probing force lower than 0.50 N does not, on average, reach the apical end of the junctional epithelium.

- The overall results of the studies on penetration of the probe tip relative to the apical termination of the junctional epithelium indicate that probe penetration depends on such factors as probing force, probe tip diameter, probing depth and degree of gingival inflammation. In addition, variations in penetration from site to site are common.

- During examination of a patient, a probing force in excess of that found suitable in these studies may be required to perform an adequate examination of less accessible areas.

- Due to anatomical differences, probe penetration in furcation pockets may vary from that along flat surfaces. In furcations, the difficulty in following the contours of the roots with the probe tip may lead to a penetration of the tip into the connective tissue between the roots (Moriarty et al.[71]).

- Overall, bleeding on probing is related to the inflammatory state of the gingival tissues. However, bleeding on probing seems to provide less reliable information about the individual site. It has been shown that bleeding may occur in what appears to be clinically healthy conditions. Conversely, at sites with apparent histological evidence of chronic inflammation, bleeding may not occur. In addition, on a site level, bleeding on probing seems to have limited reproducibility. In an effort to compensate for these limitations inherent with the scoring system of presence or absence, the clinician may prefer to consider how easily and how much it bleeds. The apparent lack of studies in which bleeding has been graduated may be a reflection of the difficulties involved in quantifying the various degrees of bleeding.

- Ideally, a diagnostic sign such as bleeding on probing should reflect the degree of activity or chronicity of the tested lesion. It is a well-known clinical observation that some patients may demonstrate obvious inflammation of the gingival tissues and show a high bleeding tendency over a prolonged period without developing any loss of periodontal attachment. Apparently, in these individuals, the lesions are quiescent or inactive. During recent years, research has been focused on attempts at finding improved diagnostic tools for site-level use in periodontitis patients. As of yet, however, there seems to be no practical substitute for, or supplement to, bleeding on probing.

- It is somewhat surprising that suppuration on probing has received very little attention relative to disease activity in chronic periodontitis. This may possibly be explained by the fact that drainage of pus after probing can be considered to be as dependent on such factors as the anatomy of the site as it is on disease activity.

- The studies reviewed here on the reproducibility of recordings of probing depth and probing attachment level demonstrate that a deviation of ≥ 2 mm may occur for 5-10% of duplicate measurements. A similar degree of reproducibility has been observed in several other studies, such as Glavind & Löe[38], Goodson et al.[39], Cercek et al.[22], Haffajee et al.[44], Watts[95], Janssen et al.[53,55] and Best et al.[13]. For clinical purposes, this suggests that a difference amounting to 2 mm between recordings obtained at 2 different time points may not necessarily reflect a true change. The possibility of a probing error should always be considered, particularly for molars and deeper sites, where the reproducibility error is potentially of greater magnitude.

- The larger differences in duplicate recordings are probably mainly due to difficulties in reproducing the placement of the probe tip in the periodontal pocket. This problem is perhaps magnified when the attachment level has a pronounced oblique or irregular course over a given tooth surface. A slight variation in placement or angulation of the probe may give a markedly different reading under these circumstances.

- Constant force probes combined with electronic reading of the depths and direct computer input have been developed and used for research purposes. Such devices may improve the reproducibility of the recordings (Magnusson et al.[68], Marks et al.[69], Osborn et al.[75]).

- In addition to errors due to limited reproducibility of the probing measurements, the validity of probing measurements has to be considered. In this respect, the extent of penetration of the probe tip relative to histological landmarks is important. Probing differences between 2 time points may reflect fluctuations in the inflammatory status of the gingival tissues rather than connective tissue destruction due to periodontitis.

CHAPTER 3

Effect of initial periodontal treatment

A large number of studies are available on the effects of oral hygiene instruction and supra- and subgingival debridement in adult patients with various degrees of chronic periodontitis. The studies reviewed here have been selected to address the following questions:

- What amount of improvement of gingival conditions can be expected in patients with chronic periodontitis after initial periodontal therapy?

- What variations in healing response can be observed:
  - for different patients?
  - for different tooth types?
  - for teeth and lesions with different degrees of initial involvement?
  - for buccal, lingual, approximal and furcation sites?

- What is the frequency and localization of sites with continued probing attachment loss?

- What are the clinical characteristics of sites with continued probing attachment loss?

- To what extent is trauma to the periodontal tissues inflicted during subgingival instrumentation?

- Can changes in the periodontal bone height be observed from conventional radiographs as a result of initial periodontal treatment?

BADERSTEN[3] and BADERSTEN ET AL.[4,5,7,8,10] studied the effect of a combined therapy of oral hygiene instruction and supra- and subgingival instrumentation.

Subjects and procedures

- 49 patients, 28-64 years of age, with severe chronic periodontitis

- only incisors, cuspids and bicuspids included for study

- periodontal pockets 5-12 mm with subgingival calculus and bleeding on probing on 2 or more aspects of each tooth

- no limitation as to the degree of periodontal breakdown of the included teeth, apart from teeth with periodontal pockets extending to the root apex

- 6 aspects of each tooth examined; probing force: 0.75 N; probe tip diameter: 0.50 mm

- each individual provided teeth for study from either the maxilla or the mandible

- oral hygiene instruction combined with crown and root debridement under local anesthesia

- additional hygiene instruction and rubber cup polishing of teeth according to individual needs

- 24 months of observation

- analysis of results:
    - overall results for sites of different initial probing depth after a single episode of supra- and subgingival instrumentation at baseline (1368 sites in 33 of the patients)
    - frequency and localization of individual sites with loss of probing attachment level (2532 sites in all 49 patients)
    - distribution of frequency of sites with gain and loss of probing attachment level among patients (1688 approximal sites in all 49 patients)
    - frequency of gain and loss of probing attachment level relative to various clinical and radiographic characteristics (1688 approximal sites in all 49 patients)

Results
Overall results

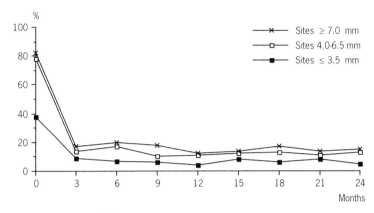

Fig. 3-1. Plaque scores throughout the 24-month observation interval for sites with different initial probing depth

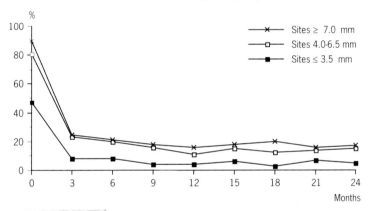

Fig. 3-2. Bleeding scores throughout the 24-month observation interval for sites with different initial probing depth

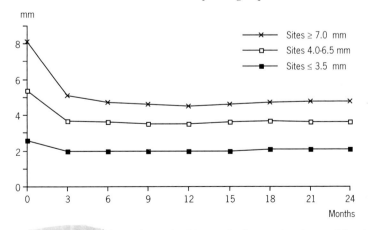

Fig. 3-3. Probing depth throughout the 24-month observation interval for sites with different initial probing depth

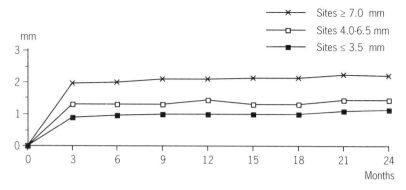

Fig. 3-4. Gingival recession throughout the 24-month observation interval for sites with different initial probing depth

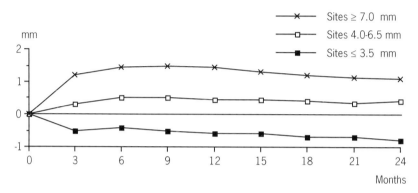

Fig. 3-5. Change of probing attachment level throughout the 24-month observation interval for sites with different initial probing depth

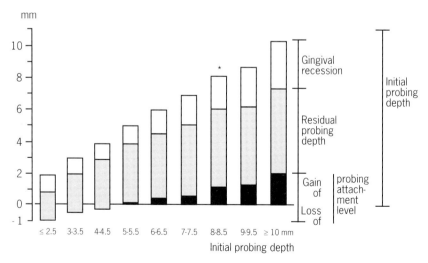

Fig. 3-6. Dimensional changes 0-24 months for sites with different initial probing depth.
* Interpretation: for sites initially 8-8.5 mm deep, gingival recession amounted to about 2 mm, gain of probing attachment 1 mm and residual probing depth 5 mm

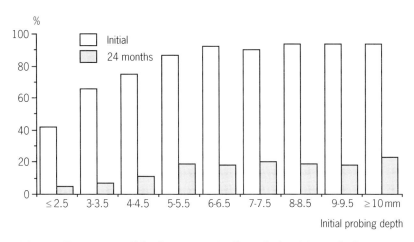

Fig. 3-7. Percentage of bleeding sites initially and after 24 months for sites with different initial probing depth

Frequency and localization of sites with probing attachment loss

Table 3-1

Percentage of sites with probing attachment loss 0-24 months by surface location and initial probing depth

	Sites with probing attachment loss*	
	Number	**Percent**
Surface location		
buccal	44	10
lingual	9	2
proximal	67	4
Initial probing depth		
≤ 3.5 mm	58	10
4.0-6.5 mm	45	4
≥ 7.0 mm	17	2
Total (n = 2532)	120	5

* Determined from the use of linear regression analysis of recordings obtained every third month. A y-axis difference ≥ 1.5 mm (= minimum loss) and $P < 0.05$ required.

Distribution of the percentage of sites with gain and loss of probing attachment level 0-24 months among patients

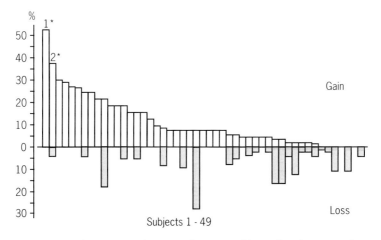

Fig. 3-8. Percentage of approximal sites with gain and loss of probing attachment level ≥ 1.5 mm (determined from linear regression analysis; see page 12) for each of 49 subjects sorted by their percentage of sites with gain of probing attachment. *Interpretation: subject 1 shows 52% of sites with gain and 0% with loss. Subject 2 shows 37% of sites with gain and 4% with loss of probing attachment

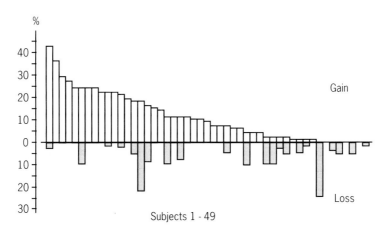

Fig. 3-9. Percentage of approximal sites with gain and loss of probing attachment level ≥ 1.5 mm (determined from end-point analysis using the gap method; see page 11) for each of 49 subjects sorted by their percentage of sites with gain of probing attachment

Note: The subjects are not sorted in the same manner in the above 2 figures since probing attachment loss has been determined with different methods.

Percentage of sites with gain and loss of probing attachment level 0-24 months relative to various clinical and radiographic characteristics

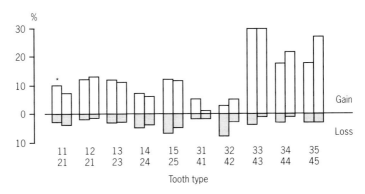

Fig. 3-10. Percentage of approximal sites with gain and loss of probing attachment level ≥ 1.5 mm determined from both linear regression analysis (left side of each paired bar) and end-point analysis (right side of each paired bar) for different tooth types. *Interpretation: for maxillary central incisors (11, 21), 10% of sites show gain and 3% show loss as determined with regression analysis; 8% show gain and 4% show loss as determined with end-point analysis

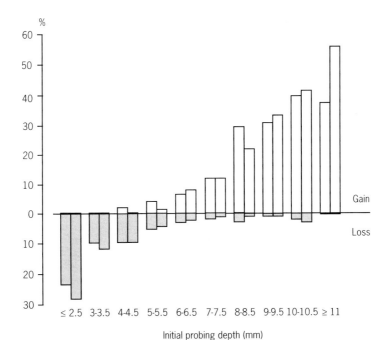

Fig. 3-11. Percentage of approximal sites with gain and loss of probing attachment level ≥ 1.5 mm determined from both linear regression analysis (left side of each paired bar) and end-point analysis (right side of each paired bar) for surfaces with different initial probing depth

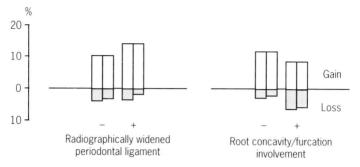

Fig. 3-12. Percentage of approximal sites with gain and loss of probing attachment level ≥ 1.5 mm determined from both linear regression analysis (left side of each paired bar) and end-point analysis (right side of each paired bar) for surfaces with and without radiographically widened periodontal ligament at 0 months and surfaces without and with root concavity/furcation involvement

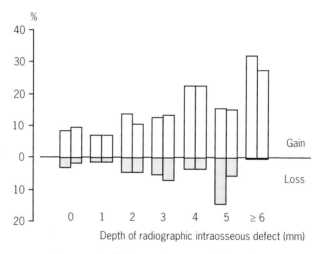

Fig. 3-13. Percentage of approximal sites with gain and loss of probing attachment level ≥ 1.5 mm determined from both linear regression analysis (left side of each paired bar) and end-point analysis (right side of each paired bar) for surfaces with different depths of radiographic intraosseous defect

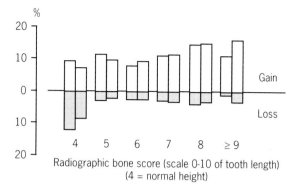

Fig. 3-14. Percentage of approximal sites with gain and loss of probing attachment level ≥ 1.5 mm determined from both linear regression analysis (left side of each paired bar) and end-point analysis (right side of each paired bar) for surfaces with different periodontal bone height

Comments

- On average, the healing following initial periodontal therapy appeared almost complete at 3 months following debridement.

- More gingival recession was obtained in deeper than in shallower sites. This is to be expected, as the amount of recession will reflect the bulk of inflamed tissue initially.

- More gain of probing attachment was obtained in deeper than in shallower sites. The amount of re-adaptation of tissues at the apical aspect of the pocket seems to relate to the height of the soft tissues initially. Deeper sites may heal with a greater amount of adaptation of the pocket lining to the root surface or with a less penetrable junctional epithelium.

- Bleeding scores were reduced to 15-20% irrespective of initial pocket depth. These results, together with the marked probing changes in the deeper sites, indicate that there is no certain magnitude of initial pocket depth wherein initial periodontal therapy is not effective. It should also be kept in mind that these results were obtained after a single episode of debridement at baseline, followed by supragingival polishing only during the 24-month interval.

- An average loss of attachment occurred for sites with shallow initial depth. Also, the highest proportion of sites with probing attachment loss was found for sites with initial probing depth ≤ 3.5 mm and for buccal surfaces. The cause of this loss in these sites, the majority of which would seem healthy, is incompletely understood, but is elucidated in the studies by Claffey et al.[27], Claffey[25] and Claffey & Egelberg[26] (see pages 81-89).

- The results from the subgroup of sites initially ≥ 7.0 mm indicate that progression of disease can be prevented in the vast majority of these sites (note: 24 months of observation only; molar teeth not included; compare Claffey et al.[29], page 75).

- Among the 49 individuals, 2 patients demonstrated probing attachment loss for 20-30% of the approximal sites.

- The results of the distribution of gaining and losing sites among patients indicate that, for some subjects with higher proportions of approximal sites showing probing attachment gain, sites with probing attachment loss seemed to be less common, and vice versa.

- Approximal sites with probing attachment gain seemed to occur more frequently for mandibular cuspids and bicuspids than for other single-rooted teeth. The anatomy in this mandibular area may favor approximal adaptation of the gingival tissues.

- More approximal sites with probing attachment gain were seen in deeper than in shallower intraosseous defects. This is most likely explained by the fact that deeper defects are associated with deeper initial probing depth.

- A higher proportion of sites from teeth with a radiographically widened periodontal ligament at baseline, indicative of increased tooth mobility, showed probing attachment gain than teeth without such widening. This finding is probably also a reflection of the deeper initial probing depths for these mobile teeth.

- The presence of approximal root concavity or furcation involvement was associated with a lower frequency of sites with probing attachment gain and a higher frequency of sites with probing attachment loss. This could be related to difficulties in achieving adequate debridement. It could also be related to compromised adaptation of gingival tissues at concave tooth surfaces.

- Linear regression analysis and end-point gap analysis, both using a minimum difference of 1.5 mm, selected approximately the same number of sites with probing attachment change. However, only about half the sites selected by one of the methods were also identified by the other method (data not shown here). In spite of these differences in site selection, similar relationships between clinical and radiographic characteristics and probing attachment change were observed for both methods.

- None of the 49 subjects lost any of the nonmolar teeth under observation during the 24-month study period.

CLAFFEY ET AL.[29] studied the effect of initial periodontal therapy in a 42-month follow-up.

Subjects and procedures

- 17 patients, 32-65 years of age, 6 women and 11 men, with advanced chronic periodontitis (12 of these subjects are included among the cases presented in Chapters 5 and 6: Case reports, see pages 129-197)

- no periodontal treatment within the preceding 5 years

- average number of remaining teeth: 21.4

- no limitation as to the degree of periodontal breakdown of the included teeth, apart from teeth with periodontal pockets extending to the root apex

- oral hygiene instruction and a single episode of supra- and subgingival debridement under local anesthesia at baseline

- maintenance care with reinforcement of oral hygiene, debridement of deep and/or bleeding sites together with tooth polishing at varying frequencies during the observation interval (average: 2 times yearly)

- 42 months of observation

- examination at 6 sites per tooth for nonmolar teeth, 8 sites per tooth for maxillary molars and 10 sites per tooth for mandibular molars (in order to include furcation sites and buccal and lingual sites of all roots, see page 130); total of 2121 sites

- probing force: 0.50 N; probe tip diameter: 0.40 mm

- analysis of mean results of plaque, bleeding and probing measurements for:
    - nonmolar teeth
    - molar teeth

    - buccal sites (excluding furcation sites)
    - lingual sites (excluding furcation sites)
    - approximal sites (excluding furcation sites)
    - furcation sites (irrespective of surface location)

    - sites initially ≤ 3.5 mm deep
    - sites initially 4.0-6.5 mm deep
    - sites initially ≥ 7.0 mm deep

- analysis of the frequency and localization of sites with continued probing attachment loss

Results

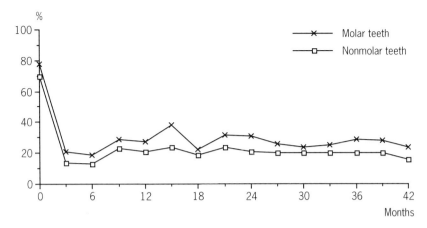

Fig. 3-15. Plaque scores throughout the 42-month observation interval for nonmolar and molar sites

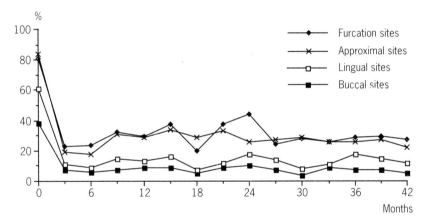

Fig. 3-16. Plaque scores throughout the 42-month observation interval for sites with different surface location

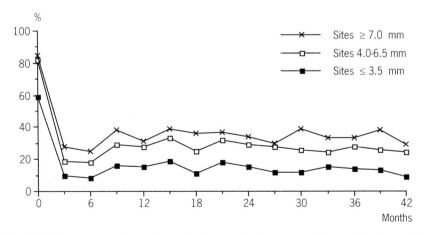

Fig. 3-17. Plaque scores throughout the 42-month observation interval for sites with different initial probing depth

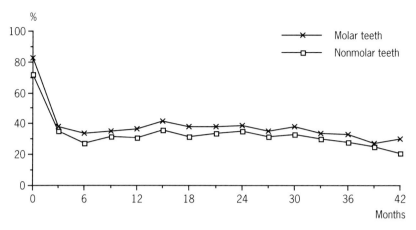

Fig. 3-18. Bleeding scores throughout the 42-month observation interval for nonmolar and molar sites

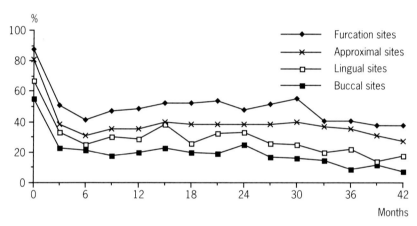

Fig. 3-19. Bleeding scores throughout the 42-month observation interval for sites with different surface location

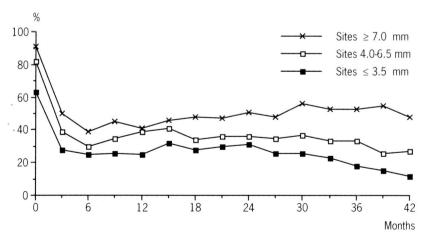

Fig. 3-20. Bleeding scores throughout the 42-month observation interval for sites with different initial probing depth

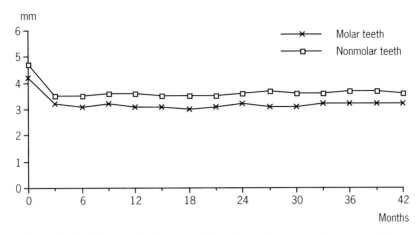

Fig. 3-21. Probing depth throughout the 42-month observation interval for nonmolar and molar sites

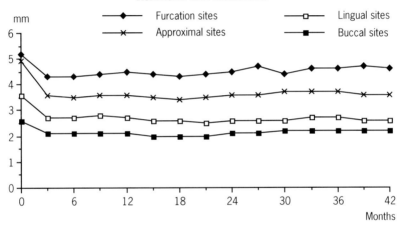

Fig. 3-22. Probing depth throughout the 42-month observation interval for sites with different surface location

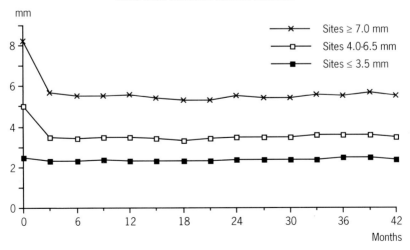

Fig. 3-23. Probing depth throughout the 42-month observation interval for sites with different initial probing depth

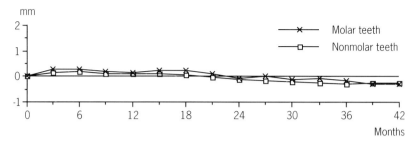

Fig. 3-24. Change of probing attachment level througout the 42-month observation interval for nonmolar and molar sites

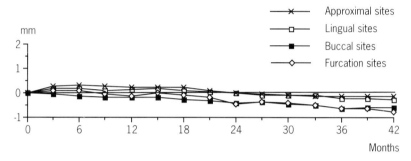

Fig. 3-25. Change of probing attachment level throughout the 42-month observation interval for sites with different surface location

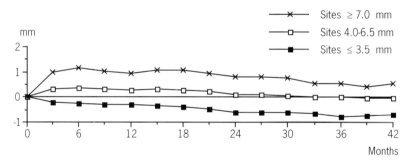

Fig. 3-26. Change of probing attachment level throughout the 42-month observation interval for sites with different initial probing depth

Table 3-2

Percentage of sites with probing attachment loss 0-42 months* by initial probing depth and surface location for each of the subjects

Sub-ject	Initial probing depth			Surface location				All sites
	≤ 3.5 mm	4.0-6.5 mm	≥ 7.0 mm	buccal	lingual	approximal	furcation	
1**	3***	0	0	4	4	0	0	1
2	3	2	4	0	0	4	0	2
3	3	0	17	22	0	3	-****	6
4	4	2	23	3	3	6	10	6
5	10	0	6	0	19	4	13	6
6	10	3	0	22	6	2	13	7
7	11	6	0	6	6	8	20	8
8	6	2	50	0	5	8	100	8
9	3	3	23	5	10	7	14	8
10	14	6	0	13	21	7	0	9
11	15	4	14	25	11	5	10	10
12	20	6	0	13	13	17	0	13
13	12	19	13	5	24	15	25	16
14	32	11	0	27	21	14	25	18
15	13	16	43	22	24	13	40	19
16	8	28	43	5	14	24	33	20
17	24	13	27	14	14	22	38	21
Mean	11	7	16	11	11	9	22	10

*   Determined from the use of linear regression analysis of recordings obtained every third month. A y-axis difference ≥1.5 mm (= minimum loss) and P<0.05 required.

**   Subjects listed according to the percentage of sites with probing attachment loss for all sites (right column).

***   Some of the percentage values in the table are based on only a few sites available from that particular category in the patient.

****   No furcation sites available.

Table 3-3
Number of subjects with tooth loss during the 42-month observation interval

Number of subjects	Number of teeth lost
12	0
4	1
1	2

Comments

- After initial improvement, the mean plaque and bleeding scores remained somewhat higher for molar teeth than for nonmolar teeth; for furcation and approximal sites than for buccal and lingual sites; and for initially deep sites than for shallower sites.

- The improvements of plaque and bleeding scores for nonmolar sites in these patients were somewhat less than those of the subjects of Badersten et al.[3] (see page 60).

- The probing depth data also varied with tooth type, surface location and initial probing depth.

- Overall, the probing attachment level recordings demonstrated a slight but gradual loss of mean attachment during the 42 months of observation. Similar to the findings by Badersten et al.[3], an average loss of attachment occurred for sites with shallow depth (see page 61).

- The frequency of individual sites with probing attachment loss during the 42-month observation interval varied among the participating 17 patients. This was seen for all sites present in a subject as well as for subgroups of sites with different initial probing depth and surface location. Overall, the highest rate of continuous deterioration was observed for furcation sites (compare Nordland et al.[72], page 78).

- This study may constitute a realistic representation of what can be achieved in clinical practice. The mean data primarily indicate successful outcome over the 42 months of observation. However, on a site basis there are signs of continuous deterioration in many of the patients.

- In addition, the results presented should be interpreted while keeping in mind that 6 (1.8%) of the total of 338 teeth available for study were lost at various points during the 42-month observation period due to progressive periodontal disease. Another 4 teeth with progression (2 patients with each 2 teeth) were subjected to surgical treatment. None of these 10 teeth were included in the data analysis. (The clinical characteristics of the teeth lost during the 42-month period are presented in Chapter 6: Case reports – tooth loss, see pages 177-197.)

- Most of the participating patients had a history of irregular dental care and presented with severely advanced chronic periodontitis. (See individual patient data and radiographs in Chapters 5 and 6: Case reports, see pages 129-197.)

(During preparation of this book, the data analysis for the above study was extended as compared with that presented in the publication by Claffey et al.[29].)

NORDLAND ET AL.[72] compared the effect of nonsurgical periodontal therapy in nonmolar sites, molar flat surfaces and molar furcations.

Subjects and procedures

- 19 patients, 29-68 years of age, with moderate to severe periodontitis

- periodontal pockets up to 12 mm deep

- a total of 2474 sites from nonmolar teeth, molar flat surfaces and molar furcations (221 molar furcation sites)

- initial oral hygiene instruction, reinforced according to individual needs at 3 and 6 months

- a single episode of supra- and subgingival debridement under local anesthesia

- probing force: 0.50 N; probe tip diameter: 0.40 mm

- 24 months of observation

- analysis of results for subgroups of furcation sites with different initial probing depth (only sites ≥ 7 mm presented here); degree of furcation involvement not recorded

Results

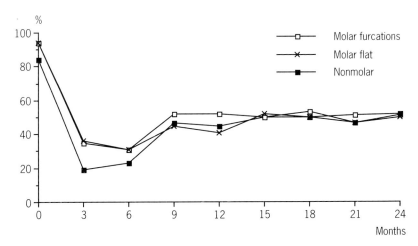

Fig. 3-27. Sites ≥ 7 mm. Plaque scores throughout the 24-month observation interval for sites with different surface location

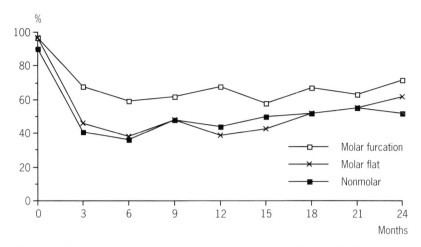

Fig. 3-28. Sites ≥ 7 mm. Bleeding scores throughout the 24-month observation interval for sites with different surface location

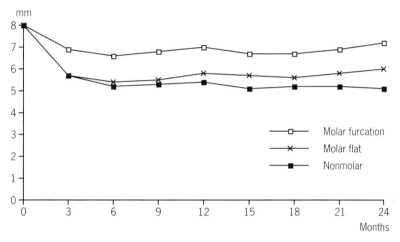

Fig. 3-29. Sites ≥ 7 mm. Probing depth throughout the 24-month observation interval for sites with different surface location

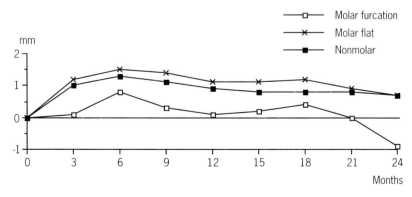

Fig. 3-30. Sites ≥ 7 mm. Change of probing attachment level throughout the 24-month observation interval for sites with different surface location

Table 3-4

Percentage of sites with probing attachment loss 0-24 months* by initial probing depth and surface location

Initial probing depth	Nonmolar sites	Molar flat surfaces	Molar furcations
≤ 3.5 mm	10	10	6
4.0-6.5 mm	4	6	12
≥ 7 mm	11	8	21
All sites	8	7	13

* Determined from the use of linear regression analysis of recordings obtained every third month. A y-axis difference ≥ 1.5 mm (= minimum loss) and $P < 0.05$ required.

Comments

- Plaque scores showed a subsequent relapse after significant improvement during the initial 6 months of observation. The plaque scores were similar for the 3 groups of sites.

- Similar to the plaque scores, relapses of the bleeding scores and the gains of probing attachment could be observed.

- Nonmolar sites and molar flat surfaces healed comparably.

- Molar furcations, on the average, demonstrated impaired healing as compared with nonmolar sites and molar flat surfaces.

- Molar furcations also showed a higher frequency of sites with probing attachment loss than the other groups of sites.

- The difference in healing response between molar furcations and other locations was most noticeable for sites ≥7 mm. Sites with shallower initial depth showed little or no variation of healing for the various locations (data not presented here). It can be assumed that most furcation sites initially ≥ 7 mm deep probably have furcation involvement, which may explain the limited healing for these areas.

- The results of this study were confirmed in a similar 2-year follow-up by Loos et al.[67]. Also, Claffey et al.[29] found impaired healing of furcation sites as compared with other site locations (see pages 70-77).

- The level of plaque control and the healing response for nonmolar sites ≥ 7.0 mm was less than that of the corresponding sites for the subjects of Badersten[3] (see pages 60-61).

CLAFFEY ET AL.[27] and CLAFFEY[25] studied the amount of probing attachment loss occurring as a result of trauma during subgingival instrumentation.

Subjects and procedures

- 9 adult periodontitis patients, 32-62 years of age

- a total of 1248 sites

- oral hygiene instruction 4 weeks prior to debridement

- a single episode of crown and root debridement under local anesthesia

- 1 operator using ultrasonic instruments (Cavitron®-Dentsply®, TFI-10 tip, maximum power setting)

- triplicate probing attachment level measurements by 3 independent examiners at 5 time points:
    - immediately preinstrumentation
    - immediately postinstrumentation
    - 3 months
    - 12 months
    - 24 months

- probing force: 0.50 N; probe tip diameter: 0.40 mm

- sites with probing attachment loss identified from the triplicate recordings using a site-specific standard deviation for measurement variability; minimal threshold for attachment loss: ≥ 1.0 mm, $P < 0.05$

- 12 months of observation (all 9 patients)

- 24 months of observation (7 patients)

Results
Mean longitudinal results

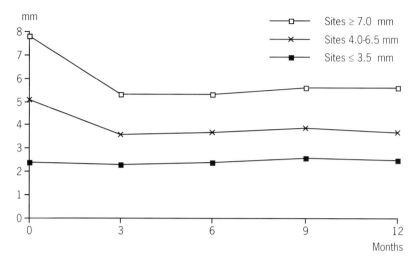

Fig. 3-31. Probing depth during 12 months of observation for sites with different initial probing depth

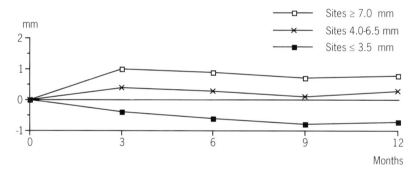

Fig. 3-32. Change of probing attachment level during 12 months of observation for sites with different initial probing depth

Means of triplicate probing attachment level measurements

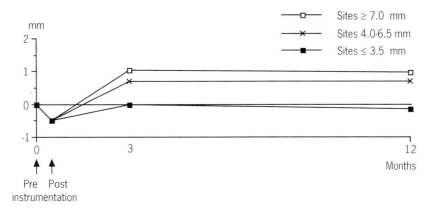

Fig. 3-33. Sites ≤ 3.5, 4.0-6.5 and ≥ 7.0 mm. Change of probing attachment level pre- to postinstrumentation and after 3 and 12 months

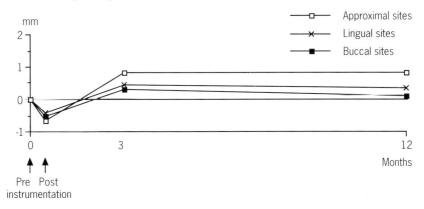

Fig. 3-34. Buccal, lingual and approximal sites. Change of probing attachment level pre- to postinstrumentation and after 3 and 12 months

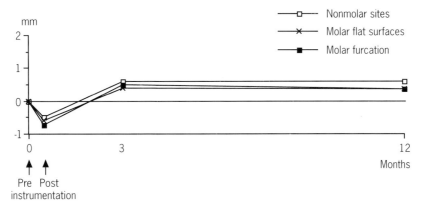

Fig. 3-35. Nonmolar sites, molar flat surfaces and molar furcation sites. Change of probing attachment level pre- to postinstrumentation and after 3 and 12 months

Table 3-5

Percentage of sites with statistically significant probing attachment loss
0-24 months ($\geq$ 1.0 mm, $P < 0.05$) during various intervals by initial probing depth

Initial probing depth (mm)	Intervals compared		
	Pre- to post-instrumentation	Pre- to 24 months	Pre- to post- *and* pre- to 24 months
$\leq$ 3.5	19	18	5
4.0-6.5	29	8	4
$\geq$7.0	25	11	4
All sites (n = 938)	24	12	4

Pre- to post = sites that lost attachment due to instrumentation.
Pre- to 24 months = sites with loss from the preinstrumentation recording to the 24-month time point.
Pre- to post **and** pre- to 24 months = sites with loss due to instrumentation that did not rebound during the subsequent 24 months.

Table 3-6

Bleeding frequency and distribution of 47 sites that lost attachment postinstrumentation to 24 months
(sites with loss subsequent to instrumentation) by initial probing depth and surface location

Initial probing depth (mm)	Bleeding frequency*	Surface location		
		Buccal/lingual	Approximal	Furcation
$\leq$ 3.5 (n = 27)	2/9	22	0	5
4.0-6.5 (n = 11)	5/9	3	4	4
$\geq$ 7.0 (n = 9)	7/9	2	3	4

* Average number of examinations at which the score was positive over the 9 examinations possible (recordings every third month).

Comments

- The mean longitudinal changes of probing depths and probing attachment levels compare well with other studies on initial periodontal therapy.

- The mean data from the triplicate probing attachment level measurements demonstrate that the instrumentation caused an average loss of probing attachment of approximately 0.5 mm. This loss occurred for all categories of initial depth and for all site locations. Similar results were obtained in a study by Nylund & Egelberg[73].

- Identification of sites with attachment loss ≥ 1.0 mm immediately following instrumentation resulted in an overall incidence of 24%.

- Rebound of the inflicted probing attachment loss was most obvious in sites initially ≥ 7.0 mm and limited in sites initially ≤ 3.5 mm. This is probably related to variation in the available gingival tissue height offering resistance to probe penetration following healing (see Badersten et al.[10], page 67).

- On the average, 12% of sites showed probing attachment loss pre- to 24 months. One third of these (4%) were sites that lost attachment during instrumentation and did not rebound during the subsequent 24 months.

- The bleeding frequency, initial probing depth and surface localization for the sites that lost probing attachment from postinstrumentation to 24 months ($n = 47$) may suggest that the loss for many of these sites was not due to a periodontal disease process.

- The results of these studies, albeit in a small number of subjects, highlight the following issues:
    - Only a small proportion of sites may show probing attachment loss due to inflammatory periodontal disease of microbial origin over a 2-year period following initial treatment (compare Claffey & Egelberg[26], pages 86-89).
    - Probing measurements postinstrumentation may be more appropriate for use as baseline recordings in longitudinal clinical studies attempting to identify diseased sites than the use of preinstrumentation measurements.

- This clinical study does not answer any questions about the histological nature of the instrumentation trauma. Is the loss of probing attachment related to injury of the coronal part of the connective tissue attachment? Is the loss merely a reflection of expansion of the gingival tissues during instrumentation, thereby facilitating probe penetration after treatment? As yet, these questions cannot be answered.

CLAFFEY & EGELBERG[26] studied the clinical characteristics of sites with probing attachment loss following initial periodontal therapy.

Subjects and procedures

- 16 patients with advanced chronic periodontitis (16 of the 17 patients included in the study reviewed on pages 70-77; see page 70 for additional details; 1 patient excluded due to lack of data from examinations necessary for the present analysis)

- criteria for identification of sites with probing attachment loss 0-42 months:
    - linear regression analysis of measurements obtained every third month; threshold for loss ≥ 1.5 mm, $P < 0.05$
    - max/min gap method, comparing 0/3 months to 39/42 months; threshold for loss ≥ 1.5 mm between deepest of 0 and 3 months and shallowest of recordings at 39 and 42 months
    - 0-month level compared with 42 months; threshold for loss ≥ 2.5 mm
    - sites satisfying all above 3 methods

- sites with probing attachment loss subgrouped with respect to:
    - surface location (buccal, lingual, approximal, furcation)
    - initial probing depth (≤ 3.5 mm, 4.0-6.5 mm, ≥ 7 mm)
    - increase in probing depth (yes/no; determined with the 3 methods as for probing attachment loss)
    - bleeding frequency (number of examinations with bleeding, 3-42 months; maximum 14)
    - suppuration on probing at any examination, 3-42 months

- criteria for identification of sites with probing attachment loss but with "questionable periodontitis" (arbitrary classification of deterioration that may not be periodontal disease of microbial origin):
    - 42-month probing depth ≤ 3.5 mm
    - bleeding on probing at ≤ 5 of 14 examinations, 3-42 months
    - no suppuration on probing at any of 14 examinations, 3-42 months

Results

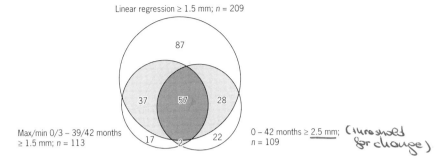

Fig. 3-36. Agreement between 3 methods for selection of sites with probing attachment loss

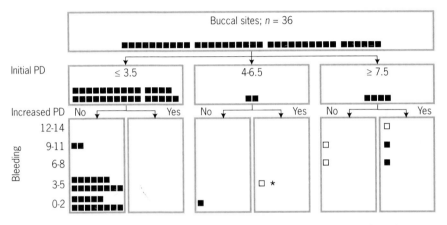

Fig. 3-37 to 3-40. Buccal, lingual, approximal and furcation sites with probing attachment loss (determined from regression analysis; threshold ≥ 1.5 mm, $P < 0.05$) by initial probing depth, increase in probing depth, bleeding and suppuration on probing.
*Interpretation: this particular site had initial probing depth (PD) between 4-6.5 mm, increased in probing depth 0-42 months, bled at 3-5 of the 14 examinations 3-42 months and showed suppuration at ≥ 1 of these examinations (filled squares = no suppuration 3-42 months)

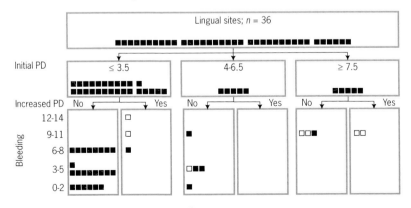

Fig. 3-38.

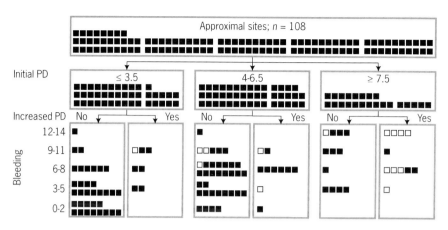

Fig. 3-39.

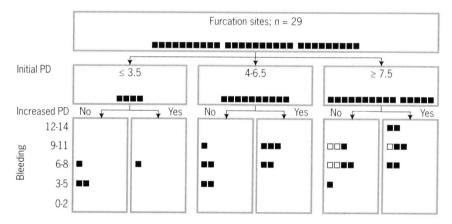

Fig. 3-40.

Table 3-7

Percentage of sites with "questionable periodontitis"* by surface location and method for identification of probing attachment loss

Surface location	Linear regression ≥ 1.5 mm	Max/min ≥ 1.5 mm	0-42 months ≥ 2.5 mm	All 3 methods
Buccal	72	69	56	55
Lingual	47	39	35	25
Approximal	27	19	20	12
Furcation	7	6	6	8
Total	35	33	26	21

* Sites ≤ 3.5 mm deep at 42 months, with bleeding on probing at ≤ 5 of 14 examinations 3-42 months and with no suppuration 3-42 months.

Comments

- Agreement between the 3 methods to determine probing attachment loss was limited. However, similar trends were seen for the characteristics of losing sites irrespective of selection method, including sites satisfying all 3 methods (data not shown here).

- High proportions of buccal and lingual sites with probing attachment loss were initially ≤ 3.5 mm deep, showed no increase in depth over the 42 months of observation and bled on probing at few of the 14 examinations between 3-42 months.

- Among approximal sites with attachment loss, increase in probing depth and frequent bleeding was more common. Yet, many sites showed no increase in depth and infrequent bleeding.

- Among furcation sites with attachment loss, increase in probing depth and frequent bleeding was proportionately more common than for buccal, lingual and approximal sites.

- When suppuration occurred, it was most often observed for initially deep sites that deepened during 0-42 months.

- This study demonstrates that sites with probing attachment loss may or may not display the clinical characteristics commonly associated with periodontitis: deepened probing depth, increased bleeding tendency and possibly suppuration.

- A classification into "questionable periodontitis" was employed (deterioration that may not be periodontal disease of microbial origin). It was found that 21-35% of all sites with attachment loss fell into this category.

- The authors speculate as to the cause of probing attachment loss for the "questionable periodontitis" sites. The following conjectural reasons were suggested: trauma from instrumentation during initial treatment and during maintenance treatment; trauma from toothbrushing and other home care procedures; remodelling of the marginal periodontal tissues as an effect of the improved and changed conditions after treatment; a gradual recession of the periodontal tissues related to the aging process; and remodelling of the periodontal structures associated with a process of continuous eruption of the teeth. However, the possibility exists that periodontitis of microbial origin can occur in the absence of pronounced clinical signs of disease.

ISIDOR ET AL.[51] studied the effect of initial treatment on the periodontal bone height during a 12-month observation period.

Subjects and procedures

- 16 patients, 28-52 years of age, with advanced periodontitis

- maxillary and mandibular incisors, cuspids and bicuspids; probing depth ≥ 5 mm on at least 1 surface of each tooth

- oral hygiene instruction and root planing under local anesthesia at baseline; maintenance care using professional tooth cleaning every second week

- full-mouth periapical radiographs at baseline and 12 months using the bisecting angle technique

- measurements of the periodontal bone height for a total of 122 approximal sites, expressed as the percentage of normal bone height (the distance from the apex of the tooth to a level 1 mm apical to the cementoenamel junction); measurements to the nearest 5% using a transparent ruler

- analysis of difference in bone height 0-12 months for each site

- reproducibility of the radiographic method evaluated from a separate set of duplicate radiographs ("1 mesial and 1 distal angulation") obtained from 1-2 teeth in each individual

Results

Table 3-8
Percentage of sites with various magnitudes of difference between duplicate radiographic recordings

Difference between duplicate recordings	% sites
0%	50
± 5% *	32
± 10% **	16
± 15% ***	2

* Corresponds to approximately 0.7 mm.
** Corresponds to approximately 1.4 mm.
*** Corresponds to approximately 2.1 mm.

90

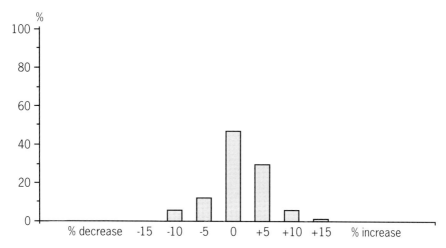

Fig. 3-41. Percentage of sites with various magnitudes of change in radiographic periodontal bone height, 0-12 months

Comments

- The result of the reproducibility test showed that variations in periodontal bone height amounting to 1-2 mm may often be recorded. These findings, however, should be interpreted in view of the deliberate use of 1 mesial and 1 distal angulation for the duplicate set of radiographs.

- Following initial periodontal treatment, somewhat more sites showed 5% gain in bone height than 5% loss in bone height. Apart from this, the results demonstrated frequencies of changes (increase and decrease) similar to those observed for the reproducibility test. This suggests that conventional radiographic techniques may not allow detection of minor bone height changes that may take place after initial periodontal therapy.

- The authors performed separate analyses for approximal sites with horizontal bone loss ($n=109$) and sites with intraosseous defects ($n=13$) but observed no difference in radiographic results (data not shown here).

BADERSTEN ET AL.[12] studied the effect of initial treatment on the periodontal bone height during a 24-month observation period.

Subjects and procedures

- 12 patients with severe chronic periodontitis (from the pool of 49 subjects of Badersten[3]; see page 60)

- maxillary and mandibular incisors, cuspids and bicuspids

- periodontal pockets 5-12 mm with subgingival calculus and bleeding on probing on 2 or more aspects of each tooth

- no limitation as to the degree of periodontal breakdown of the included teeth, apart from teeth with periodontal pockets extending to the root apex

- each individual provided teeth for study from either the maxilla or the mandible

- oral hygiene instruction together with crown and root debridement under local anesthesia

- additional hygiene instruction and rubber cup polishing of teeth at individual needs

- radiographs at baseline and 24 months obtained with a projection perpendicular to the long axis of the tooth

- identical projection for both time points ascertained by use of individual bite blocks and film holders mounted to the X-ray tube

- radiographic measurements of blinded and coded films by 1 examiner under $\times$ 10 magnification with simultaneous projection of 0- and 24-month radiographs to facilitate identification of landmarks for measurements

- all measurements repeated by the same examiner after an interval of 2 weeks

- total of 160 measurable approximal sites from 92 teeth with varying degrees and patterns of bone loss

- analysis as follows:
  - changes in bone height 0-24 months for each site recorded at the first measurement session (Cm1)
  - changes in bone height 0-24 months for each site recorded at the second measurement session 2 weeks later (Cm2)
  - differences between the bone height changes recorded at the first and the second measurement sessions (Cm1 minus Cm2)

Results

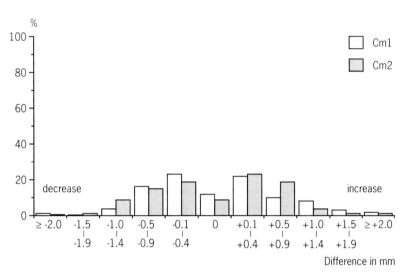

Fig. 3-42. Percentage of sites with various magnitudes of change in radiographic periodontal bone height 0-24 months

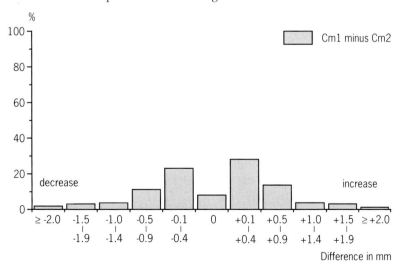

Fig. 3-43. Percentage of sites with various magnitude of difference between periodontal bone height changes 0-24 months as recorded at first and second measurement sessions

Comments

- This study was initiated during preparation of this book for the purpose of providing some additional information on the use of radiographs to evaluate the outcome of initial periodontal treatment. The 0-month radiographs were taken immediately after the baseline root planing. This allowed blinded measurements of the before-and-after pairs of radiographs due to the absence of radiographically visible calculus from the root surfaces at both time points.

- The recorded changes of periodontal bone height following treatment showed a similar distribution of sites with increase and decrease of bone level. This was true for both measurements performed by the examiner. This suggests that the recorded changes may be a reflection of measurement error rather than true bone height changes.

- The fact that the differences between changes recorded at the 2 examinations (Cm1 minus Cm2) show a distribution of sites with increase and decrease in bone level similar to that of the separate readings (Cm1) and (Cm2) seems to confirm the suspicion that measurement error is the primary cause of the recorded changes. Expressed differently: the similarity of the Cm1 minus Cm2 distribution to the individual Cm1 and Cm2 distributions indicates that the recorded Cm1 and Cm2 values are random and an expression of the measurement error.

- Thus, the results of this study, together with those of the study by Isidor et al.[51] (see pages 90-91) indicate that conventional radiographic techniques, including the use of standardized projection, do not allow detection of periodontal bone height changes of the magnitude that may take place following initial periodontal therapy. Difficulties in determination of the location of the marginal bone crest seem to cause measurement error, which precludes observation of any true change.

- Improvements following initial periodontal treatment have been observed using more advanced methods that allow measurements of minor changes in the mineral content of the marginal bone. Schmidt et al.[84] and Okano et al.[74] used subtraction radiography and Dubrez et al.[31] used a photometric technique to measure bone density. With these techniques, currently not used in clinical practice, the difficulties in assessing the location of the marginal bone crest are avoided in favor of more objective quantification of the amounts of bone minerals.

GENERAL COMMENTS

- A multitude of studies on initial periodontal therapy are available in the literature, confirming the observations reviewed in this chapter. It can be argued that the degree of success of the treatment is difficult to evaluate from most of the studies, including the ones reviewed above, as they have not included an untreated control group. However, there is little reason to believe that a chronic disease such as periodontitis would show an improvement over time without treatment. On the contrary, a gradual deterioration is to be expected (Axelsson & Lindhe[2], Lindhe et al.[61], Buckley & Crowley[18], Albandar et al.[1], Löe et al.[64], Lindhe et al.[63]).

- The studies on initial periodontal treatment reviewed in this chapter have utilized experienced operators for the subgingival debridement. Less experienced clinicians may not achieve corresponding results (Brayer et al.[16], Fleischer et al.[34]).

- The cause of the impaired healing for furcation lesions may be related to the difficulties in achieving adequate debridement of these sites (Matia et al.[70], Fleischer et al.[34]). In addition, the anatomy of the furcation area may not permit sufficient adaptation of the gingival tissues to the tooth surfaces to prevent subgingival recolonization of microorganisms after debridement (Loos et al.[66]).

- Badersten et al.[8] found that 5% of the sites demonstrated probing attachment loss ≥ 1.5 mm after 24 months as determined with regression analysis. Using the same method, Claffey et al.[29] found probing attachment loss for 10% of sites after 42 months of monitoring. In a further analysis of the 10% of sites identified after 42 months, Claffey & Egelberg[26] found that they displayed highly varying bleeding frequencies, initial probing depths and changes in probing depths over time. In treated subjects, probing attachment loss appears to take place due to reasons other than disease of microbial origin for a significant proportion of sites. Trauma from instrumentation has been demonstrated as one of these causes, but does not seem to provide the entire explanation. It seems unlikely that instrumentation trauma would be the cause of the gradual, posttreatment probing attachment loss observed most frequently amongst shallow buccal and lingual sites.

- Toothbrushing trauma is another possible source of attachment loss, especially in the light of the frequent occurrence of loss for buccal surfaces. However, loss of probing attachment also occurs for shallow sites with approximal location. Thus, it is not a phenomenon related to buccal surfaces only. This makes it less likely that toothbrushing trauma and instrumentation trauma can account for all nondisease attachment loss.

- Some indirect evidence from the studies by Claffey et al.[27] and Claffey[25] suggests that a remodelling of the periodontal tissues may occur after initial periodontal treatment (data not presented here). According to this concept, shallow sites located adjacent to deep lesions would respond to treatment with some attachment loss due to a levelling process as part of the healing response. Other conjectured sources of probing attachment loss include a gradual recession of periodontal attachment levels related to the aging process and a remodelling of the periodontal structures associated with a process of continuous eruption of the teeth.

- The analyses of the studies in this chapter included evaluations of subgroups of polarized sites with different initial probing depth: ≤ 3.5 mm and ≥ 7.0 mm. This approach reflects the desire to evaluate the therapy relative to the severity of the treated lesion. However, this type of data analysis is somewhat flawed by a statistical artifact known as regression towards the mean. Due to this phenomenon, subgroups of deep lesions will be observed as somewhat shallower on repeated measurement, even if no treatment was provided. Subgroups of shallow sites will be somewhat deeper. The artifact comes into play when the changes following therapy of a given measurement, such as probing depth, are related to their own initial value. The magnitude of this problem is related to the degree of reproducibility of the particular measurement under analysis and can be determined if the degree of reproducibility is known. For the studies by Badersten[3], it was found that the artifact may amount to about 0.2 mm for both of the 2 subgroups (≤ 3.5 mm and ≥ 7 mm). This means that the observed changes of probing depth and probing attachment level for these subgroups should be adjusted by about 0.2 mm in order to attain the true changes (Egelberg[32]). This amount of adjustment does not, however, substantially alter the overall outcome.

- Several studies are available comparing initial periodontal therapy to various types of surgical treatment. So far, these studies have failed to demonstrate an advantage of surgical procedures over nonsurgical therapy (see Egelberg[33]).

CHAPTER 4

Prediction and evaluation of deterioration

Ideally, a clinician would like to be able to predict the outcome of treatment prior to therapy. Subsequent to treatment, there is a need to evaluate the effectiveness of the procedures used. Prediction and evaluation, in order to be comprehensive, should be carried out on a patient level as well as on an individual tooth and site level.

In spite of the difficulties involved with this type of research, investigators have attempted to clarify some of the problems. The studies reviewed here address the following questions:

- What baseline clinical markers are related to subsequent periodontal deterioration?

- Can experienced clinicians predict the lack of effectiveness of initial periodontal treatment on an individual site basis?

- To what extent are deeper residual probing depths, present at re-evaluation a number of months after initial treatment, an indication of lack of effect of treatment?

- To what extent do scores of plaque, bleeding on probing, suppuration on probing and probing depth, recorded from individual sites at regular intervals after initial treatment, relate to continuous periodontal deterioration?

LINDHE ET AL.[62] and HAFFAJEE ET AL.[45] examined the relationship between various baseline conditions and subsequent probing attachment loss over a 24-month period in untreated subjects.

Subjects and procedures

- 265 subjects from a random sample of 20- to 79-year-old individuals of a city population

- no periodontal therapy during 24 months of observation

- examinations at baseline, after 12 months and after 24 months

- mean baseline approximal probing depth for nonmolar teeth ranging from 2.5 mm for the 20- to 29-year-olds to 3.0 mm for 70- to 79-year-olds; corresponding values for molars: 3.0 and 3.7 mm respectively

- gingivitis (redness) and dental plaque along the gingival margin recorded at 4 sites per tooth

- bleeding on probing, probing depths and probing attachment levels measured at 6 sites per tooth

- criterion for probing attachment loss: sites with ≥ 3 mm loss comparing the recording at 12 or 24 months to the baseline measurement

- analyses of the association between various baseline conditions and subsequent probing attachment loss on a subject level (12-month data) and on a site level (24-month data)

Results

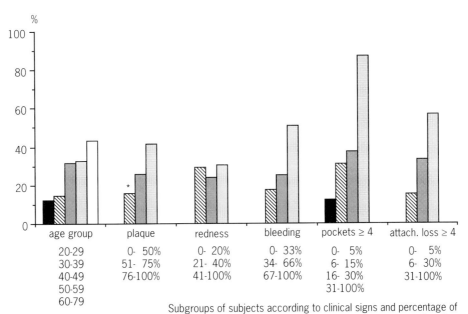

Fig. 4-1. Percentage of subjects with ≥ 1 sites with probing attachment loss 0-12 months by baseline scores.
*Interpretation: 18% of subjects with plaque scores between 0% and 50% had ≥ 1 sites with probing attachment loss ≥ 3 mm during the 12-month period

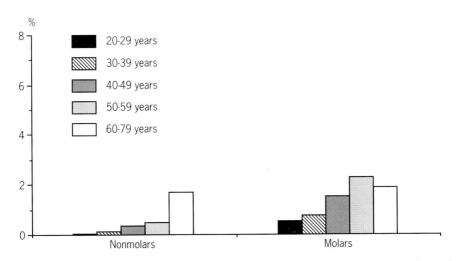

Fig. 4-2. Percentage of sites with probing attachment loss 0-24 months for nonmolar and molar teeth by age groups

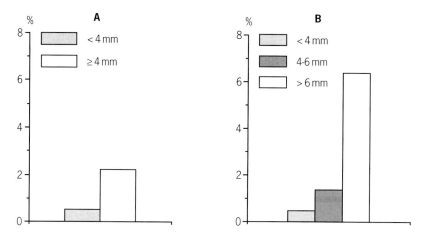

Fig. 4-3. Percentage of sites with probing attachment loss 0-24 months by initial probing depth (A) and initial attachment level (B)

Comments

- Probing attachment loss ≥ 3 mm at ≥ 1 sites was observed for 27% of the subjects after 12 months of observation and for 39% of the subjects after 24 months of monitoring.

- 0.7% of all sites showed probing attachment loss ≥ 3 mm over 24 months.

- The site-level analysis showed that the frequency of sites with probing attachment loss ≥ 3 mm:
  - increased with increasing age of the patient;
  - was higher for molars than for nonmolars; and
  - was higher for sites with increased probing depth and increased attachment loss at baseline.

- The subject-level analysis demonstrated an association between subsequent probing attachment loss at ≥ 1 sites in the dentition and baseline severity of the disease, as expressed by the percentage of sites with probing depth ≥ 4 mm and by the percentage of sites with attachment loss ≥ 4 mm. Baseline full-mouth plaque and bleeding scores were also related to subsequent attachment loss. Gingival redness did not show this relationship.

- Based on the results of statistical analysis of the patient-level data (log-linear analysis), the authors propose that the association of baseline plaque and bleeding scores to subsequent attachment loss was primarily an effect of the strong relationship of baseline plaque and bleeding scores to baseline severity of disease. Thus, baseline severity of disease, rather than baseline plaque and bleeding scores, may predict subsequent probing attachment loss.

- Although these studies demonstrate a predictive value of the baseline severity of the disease, they failed to demonstrate a predictive value for gingival redness, and they may also have failed to show a predictive value for plaque and bleeding scores.

- The low prevalence of probing attachment loss ≥ 3 mm after 24 months (0.7% of all sites) is probably explained by the fact that the group of individuals under study was a sample of a city population with little periodontal disease at baseline. This low prevalence brings out a methodological problem, as the magnitude of the prevalence is similar to the chance for a probing error of ≥ 3 mm (see studies on probing reproducibility, pages 40-45). Thus, the authors estimated that 25-50% of the sites identified with probing attachment loss ≥ 3 mm may in fact be deviations due to probing errors.

- Probing errors occur more often in deeper lesions than in shallower lesions (see page 44). Deeper lesions are more common in older than in younger individuals. Accordingly, one would expect associations similar to those observed in this study, even if the majority of sites identified with attachment loss ≥ 3 mm were due to probing errors.

- Subject-level analysis based on individuals having ≥ 2 sites with probing attachment loss ≥ 3 mm, rather than ≥ 1 sites, would reduce the possible influence of probing error. The authors reported that such analyses were performed and that the associations between baseline clinical scores and probing attachment loss were essentially unaltered. This finding lessens the concern about probing errors.

GRBIC ET AL.[41] and GRBIC & LAMSTER[40] examined the relationship between various baseline conditions and subsequent probing attachment loss over a 6-month period.

Subjects and procedures

- 75 subjects, 32-69 years of age, with chronic periodontitis

- duplicate baseline examinations, 1 week apart, followed by 1-2 h of scaling and root planing without use of local anesthesia

- duplicate final examinations after 6 months

- a total of 4 examiners (initial calibration exercises); patients examined by same examiner at 0 and 6 months

- bleeding on probing, probing depths and probing attachment levels measured at 6 sites per tooth

- criterion for probing attachment loss: sites with probing attachment loss ≥ 2.5 mm comparing means of the duplicate measurements at 6 months to the baseline means

- analysis of associations between probing attachment loss 0-6 months and various baseline conditions on a patient and site basis

Results

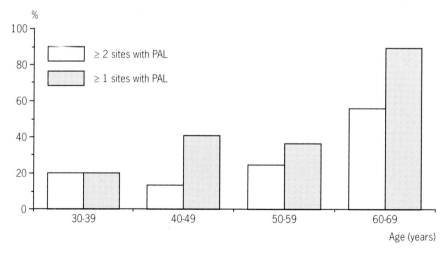

Fig. 4-4. Percentage of subjects with probing attachment loss (PAL) 0-6 months by age groups

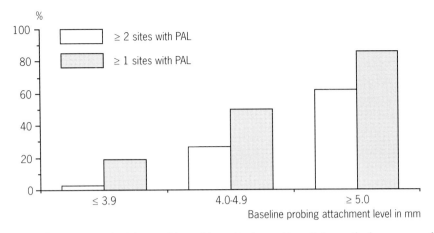

Fig. 4-5. Percentage of subjects with probing attachment loss 0-6 months by groups of baseline probing attachment level (mean baseline probing attachment level calculated for each patient)

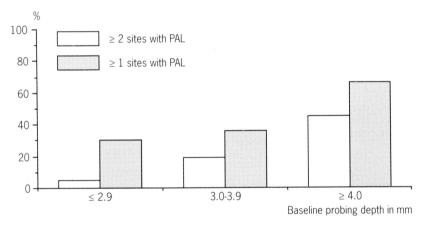

Fig. 4-6. Percentage of subjects with probing attachment loss 0-6 months by groups of baseline probing depth (mean baseline probing depth calculated for each patient)

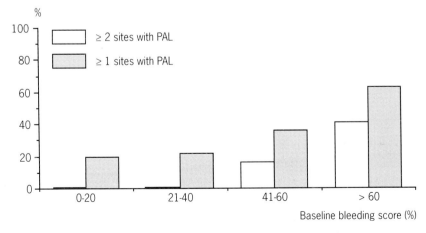

Fig. 4-7. Percentage of subjects with probing attachment loss 0-6 months by bleeding on probing groups (percentage of sites with bleeding on probing calculated for each patient)

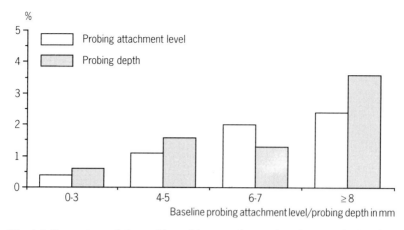

Fig. 4-8. Percentage of sites with probing attachment loss 0-6 months by their baseline probing attachment level and probing depth

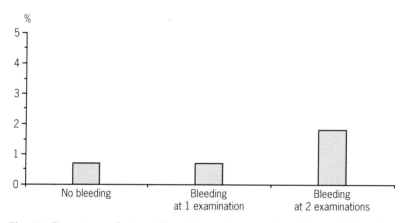

Fig. 4-9. Percentage of sites with probing attachment loss 0-6 months by their bleeding frequency at baseline examinations

Comments

- 31 of the 75 subjects (41%) showed probing attachment loss ≥ 2.5 mm at ≥ 1 sites during the 6 months of study.

- 113 of the 11,466 sites (1%) showed probing attachment loss ≥ 2.5 mm.

- On a patient level, the age of the individuals, baseline bleeding scores and baseline severity of the disease (mean probing depth and mean probing attachment loss) were related to subsequent probing attachment loss. Using statistical analysis (logistic modelling), the authors found that baseline mean probing attachment loss showed the strongest relationship to probing attachment loss 0-6 months.

- On a site level, the severity of the disease, as defined by probing depth and probing attachment level, was also related to subsequent probing attachment loss. Bleeding on probing showed a limited association with probing attachment loss 0-6 months on a site basis.

- An observation interval of 6 months seems short in the context of studying disease progression, particularly as the patients were provided with some treatment.

- The use of means of duplicate measurements together with the requirement of as much as ≥ 2.5 mm change to identify sites with probing attachment loss reduced the chance of including sites due to probing error. However, Janssen et al.[55] found that the chance of error using means of duplicate measurements and a threshold for loss of ≥ 2.5 mm was 0.3 %. This suggests that among the 1% sites identified with probing attachment loss in the above studies, a significant portion may still have been included due to probing errors. In addition, the findings of Claffey et al.[27] and Claffey[25] suggest that some of the sites in these patients, treated with scaling and root planing, may have lost probing attachment due to instrumentation trauma (see pages 81-85). The fact that local anesthesia was not used during treatment, however, may have reduced this possibility.

HALAZONETIS ET AL.[46] studied the association between various clinical parameters and probing attachment loss in untreated periodontitis patients.

Subjects and procedures

- 8 subjects with generalized, moderate to severe periodontitis, monitored prior to treatment

- examinations every second month; up to 12 months of monitoring

- recordings of gingival redness, bleeding on probing, probing depth and probing attachment level at 6 sites per tooth

- duplicate probing attachment level measurements, 1 week apart, at each examination interval

- probing attachment loss at any of the examination intervals evaluated by Student's *t*-test comparing all available recordings from each site before and after the time of examination; threshold for loss: 1.75 mm

- analysis of the relationship between various clinical conditions and probing attachment loss on a site level

Results

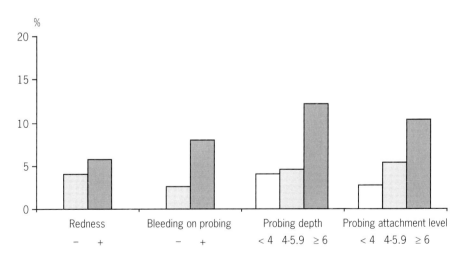

Fig. 4-10. Percentage of sites with probing attachment loss by various clinical characteristics as recorded at the visit prior to the loss

Comments

- The extent of previous involvement, as expressed by probing depth and probing attachment level, showed the strongest relationship with probing attachment loss for a given site.

- Bleeding on probing and particularly gingival redness showed limited associations with probing attachment loss.

- 5.4% of all sites showed probing attachment loss. This is a higher frequency than for the other studies mentioned above and is probably explained by the selection of subjects for study in combination with the use of a smaller threshold of change requirement.

- This study may also have sites included erroneously due to probing error. Based on the results of corresponding statistical analysis for sites with attachment gain (= 1.9% of all sites), the authors suggested that up to 25% of the selected sites could have been included due to probing errors.

JENKINS ET AL.[56] studied the association between clinical signs and probing attachment loss in periodontitis patients "resistant" to treatment.

Subjects and procedures

- 10 subjects with generalized, advanced periodontitis who had completed initial periodontal treatment with little evidence of clinical improvement (continuously high plaque scores, no reduction in bleeding scores and probing depths)

- examinations every second month during 12 months of monitoring

- no subgingival instrumentation during monitoring; supragingival scaling and polishing "as necessary"

- recordings of dental plaque, gingival redness, probing depth and probing attachment level at sites with baseline probing depth ≥ 4 mm and bleeding on probing

- sites with probing attachment loss during the 12-month observation interval identified by linear regression analysis of the recordings obtained every second month; minimum y-axis difference ≥ 1.0 mm and $P < 0.05$ required

- mean plaque and gingival redness scores calculated on a subject basis from recordings over 2-12 months

- analysis of the relationship between clinical signs and probing attachment loss on a subject level

Results

Table 4-1

Percentage of sites with probing attachment loss, mean plaque and redness scores for each of the participating subjects

Subject number	% sites with probing attachment loss	Mean Plaque Index score	Mean redness score
1	0	1.9	0.8
2	0	0.9	0.7
3	7	1.3	0.6
4	10	1.6	0.9
5	14	0.7	0.2
6	15	1.8	0.7
7	18	1.6	0.9
8	19	1.2	0.9
9	20	1.2	0.8
10	26	1.1	0.8

Table 4-2

Coefficients of correlation between mean plaque and redness scores and percentage of sites with probing attachment loss

	Coefficient of correlation
Mean Plaque Index score 2-12 months	− 0.2
Mean redness score 2-12 months	0.1

Comments

- There was quite some variation in the percentage of sites with probing attachment loss among the patients, in contrast to the limited variation in plaque and redness scores.

- Both mean plaque and redness scores showed low correlations with the percentage of sites with probing attachment loss.

- The authors performed a multitude of analyses on the relationships of probing depth, Plaque Index and redness scores to probing attachment loss (data not shown here). All of these analyses failed to demonstrate any association between the clinical signs and probing attachment loss.

- The required y-axis difference for identification of probing attachment loss using linear regression analysis was set to ≥ 1.0 mm in this study. This limited threshold may lead to inclusion of sites with questionable attachment loss. Further analysis using a difference of ≥ 1.5 mm may well have been of interest.

BOLIN ET AL.[15] examined the relationship between various baseline characteristics and periodontal bone loss over a 10-year period.

Subjects and procedures

- 406 subjects from a random sample of 18- to 65-year-old individuals in an urban population

- baseline examination included
    - Plaque and Calculus Indices (Greene & Vermillion)
    - Periodontal Index (Russell)
    - approximal alveolar bone level (periapical radiographs)
    - smoking habits (index graded 0 to 3)

- repeated radiographic examination after 10 years; bone loss during the 10-year follow-up measured as a percentage of root length

- no special provisions for treatment; dental visits and treatment at the discretion of the subjects

Results

Table 4-3
Coefficients of correlation between various baseline
characteristics and periodontal bone loss during 10 years of follow-up

Baseline characteristic	Coefficient of correlation
Baseline bone level	0.58
Periodontal Index	0.50
Calculus Index	0.39
Plaque Index	0.36
Age of individual	0.24
Smoking Index	0.15

Comments

- Although both baseline Plaque and Calculus Indices related to bone loss during the subsequent 10-year period, baseline bone level and Periodontal Index showed the strongest correlations. Similarly, in a study of radiographic bone heights in 201 subjects, Papapanou et al.[77] and Papapanou & Wennström[76] found an association between baseline bone level and bone loss during a subsequent 10-year period.

VANOOTEGHEM ET AL.[94] studied the ability of experienced clinicians to identify sites showing lack of response to treatment and continuous deterioration after initial periodontal therapy.

Subjects and procedures

- 11 subjects, 34-53 years of age, with advanced chronic periodontitis

- oral hygiene instruction at baseline, reinforced at intervals during the observation period

- an initial, single episode of supra- and subgingival debridement under local anesthesia

- maintenance care with debridement of deep and/or bleeding sites together with tooth polishing every third month, starting at 12 months

- 24 months of observation (all 11 subjects)

- 36 months of observation (6 subjects)

- evaluations by clinicians:
  - independent examinations by 3 experienced periodontists
  - records available for the clinicians: medical and dental history, full-mouth radiographs, study models, plaque scores, bleeding on probing scores and probing depths
  - each clinician asked to identify sites that they felt would not respond to initial treatment, but would continue to deteriorate and lose attachment (prediction of questionable sites)

- evaluation schedule:
  - prediction at baseline prior to therapy
  - prediction at 3 months after initial therapy (3-month scores of plaque, bleeding on probing and probing depth also available to the clinicians)

- for analysis of results, only sites identified as questionable by at least 2 of the 3 clinicians were included

- the predictions of the clinicians were evaluated against probing attachment loss after 1 year, after 2 years and after 3 years as determined from linear regression analysis of probing attachment level measurements performed every third month:
  - threshold level 1: ≥ 1.0 mm loss; $P < 0.05$
  - threshold level 2: ≥ 1.5 mm loss; $P < 0.05$

- Calculations of diagnostic predictability = the percentage of sites deemed questionable by at least 2 of the 3 clinicians that showed probing attachment loss at 12, 24 or 36 months

Results

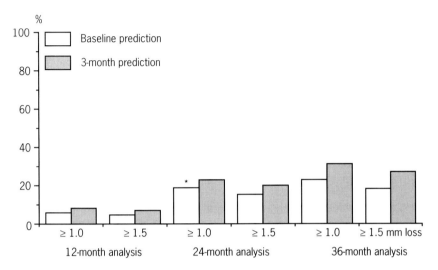

Fig. 4-11. Diagnostic predictability of questionable sites for probing attachment loss. *Interpretation: 19% of sites deemed questionable by at least 2 of the 3 clinicians at baseline showed probing attachment loss ≥ 1.0 mm after 24 months

Comments

- The diagnostic predictability at 3-month re-evaluation seemed somewhat improved compared with that at baseline.

- The clinicians' predictions improved with longer follow-up of the treatment; that is, an increasing number of sites that had been identified as questionable at baseline or at 3 months demonstrated probing attachment loss at progressive time points. This improved predictive power may, however, be explained, at least in part, by the increase in the proportion of sites with probing attachment loss with increasing time.

- Although the results indicate that the predictions were associated with subsequent probing attachment loss, the predictability amounted to a maximum of 30%. Considering that the predictions were made by experienced periodontists, and that the analyses were safeguarded by the use of sites identified by at least 2 of the 3 clinicians, the results highlight the difficulties involved in the evaluation of periodontal treatment results.

CLAFFEY ET AL.[28] studied the diagnostic value of residual probing depth following initial periodontal therapy to indicate the early response to therapy.

Subjects and procedures

- 9 patients, 36-62 years of age, with advanced chronic periodontitis and at least 10 sites with probing depth ≥ 7 mm (same subjects as those of Claffey et al.[27], see pages 81-85)

- a total of 1248 sites

- oral hygiene instruction provided during a number of sessions prior to baseline recordings

- a single episode of supra- and subgingival debridement under local anesthesia at baseline

- probing attachment levels measured in triplicate by 3 independent examiners for the purpose of determining the reproducibility of the attachment measurements for each site, and using this information to apply a threshold of ≥ 1 mm for change of probing attachment level

- probing attachment levels recorded:
  – at baseline prior to instrumentation
  – at baseline immediately after instrumentation
  – at 3 months
  – at 12 months

- 12 months of observation

- calculation of the percentage of sites with ≥ 1 mm loss, no change and ≥ 1 mm gain of probing attachment for sites of different residual probing depth at 3 and 12 months

Results

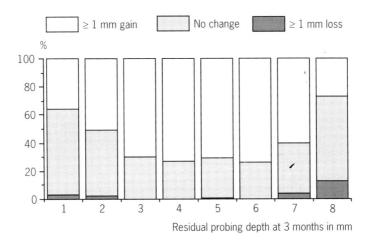

Fig. 4-12. Percentage of sites with loss, no change and gain of probing attachment from immediately postinstrumentation to 3 months by residual probing depth at 3 months

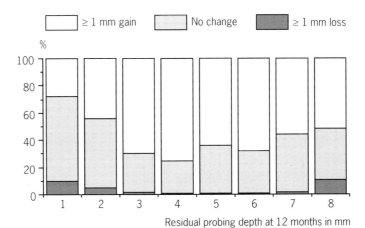

Fig. 4-13. Percentage of sites with loss, no change and gain of probing attachment from immediately postinstrumentation to 12 months by residual probing depth at 12 months

Comments

- Triplicate probing attachment level measurements at each time point and calculation of measurement variability for each site allowed the use of a change of only ≥ 1 mm to identify sites with probing attachment change without any significant risk of inclusion of sites due to probing error.

- Measurements of probing attachment level both prior to and after instrumentation demonstrated that a certain amount of probing attachment loss takes place due to trauma from instrumentation (an average of 0.5 mm: see Claffey et al.[27], page 83).

- Due to trauma inflicted from instrumentation, probing attachment levels recorded immediately after subgingival debridement may form a more appropriate baseline for determination of subsequent changes than do measurements prior to instrumentation.

- The results demonstrate that probing attachment gain ≥ 1 mm had taken place at both 3 and 12 months for 65-75% of the sites with residual probing depths of 5-6 mm and for 60-70% of the sites with residual depths of 7-8 mm.

- The frequency of probing attachment loss ≥ 1 mm was low for all subgroups of residual probing depth.

- The results indicate that a relatively deep residual probing depth 3-12 months after initial therapy, by itself, provides little evidence of lack of improvement compared with baseline. A site with deep residual probing depth may, in fact, have undergone substantial improvement in probing attachment levels compared with baseline.

BADERSTEN ET AL.[11] studied the diagnostic predictability of scores of plaque, bleeding, suppuration and probing depth for probing attachment loss during a period of 5 years after initial periodontal therapy.

Subjects and procedures

- 39 patients, 28-64 years of age with advanced chronic periodontitis (patients from the study reported on pages 60-69; individuals with 5 years of follow-up)

- only incisors, cuspids and bicuspids included for study

- initial periodontal therapy started at baseline

- only supragingival maintenance care during the initial 24 months of observation; thereafter subgingival debridement of deep and/or bleeding sites plus tooth polishing every 6 months

- clinical recordings every third month during the 0- to 24-month interval and every 6 months during the 24- to 60-month interval

- analysis of clinical signs at various intervals during the observation period to predict probing attachment loss at 60 months compared with baseline

- clinical signs: dental plaque along the gingival margin, bleeding on probing, suppuration on probing, residual probing depth and increase in probing depth

- frequency of supragingival plaque and bleeding on probing calculated for each site from presence/absence scores: percentage of positive scores of available examinations during the intervals 6-12, 6-24, 6-36, 6-48 and 6-60 months

- occurrence of suppuration calculated by adding the number of examinations with positive scores during the intervals 18-24, 18-36, 18-48 and 18-60 months (suppuration not recorded until 18 months)

- attachment loss between 0 and 60 months determined from linear regression analysis of all available attachment level measurements during the interval; threshold for loss: ≥ 1.5 mm; $P < 0.05$

- calculations of diagnostic predictability: the percentage of sites with a given clinical sign that have undergone probing attachment loss

Results

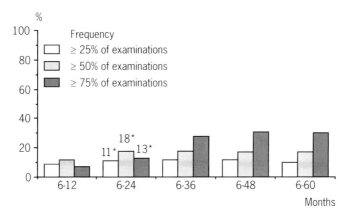

Fig. 4-14. Diagnostic predictability of plaque frequency scores.
*Interpretation: in the sites for which plaque was present in ≥ 25% of the 7 examinations
during 6-24 months, 11% demonstrated probing attachment loss during the
0- to 60-month time period; for presence ≥ 50% of the examinations, 18% lost
attachment; for presence ≥ 75% of the examinations, 13% lost attachment

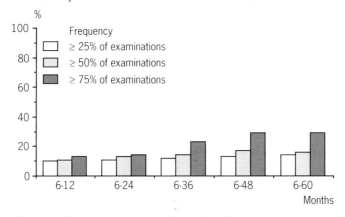

Fig. 4-15. Diagnostic predictability of bleeding frequency scores

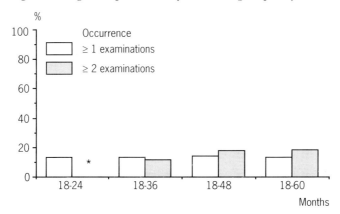

Fig. 4-16. Diagnostic predictability of suppuration frequency.
*Insufficient number of sites with suppuration available for calculation

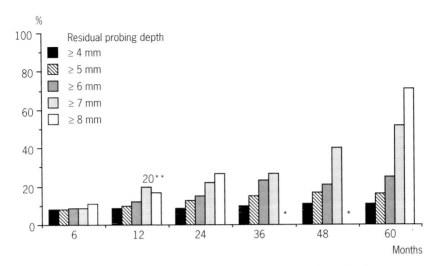

Fig. 4-17. Diagnostic predictability of residual probing depth.
*Insufficient number of sites available for calculation.
**Interpretation: for the sites that had a residual probing depth of ≥ 7 mm at
12 months, 20% demonstrated probing attachment loss during the 60 months

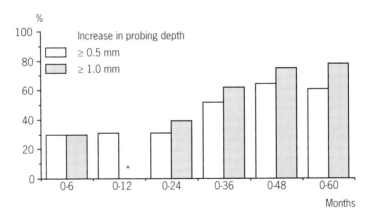

Fig. 4-18. Diagnostic predictability of increase in probing depth.
*Insufficient number of sites available for calculation

Comments

• The design and the results of this study correspond to those of the following study by Claffey et al.[29], presented on pages 120-124. The comments
for these 2 studies are combined and presented on pages 123-124.

CLAFFEY ET AL.[29] studied the diagnostic predictability of scores of plaque, bleeding, suppuration and probing depth for probing attachment loss during a period of 42 months after initial periodontal therapy.

Subjects and procedures

- 17 patients, 32-65 years of age, 6 women and 11 men, with advanced chronic periodontitis (same subjects as those reported on pages 70-77)

- oral hygiene instruction at baseline, reinforced at intervals during the observation period

- an initial, single episode of supra- and subgingival debridement under local anesthesia

- maintenance care with debridement of deep and/or bleeding sites together with tooth polishing at varying frequencies during the observation interval (average: twice yearly)

- 42 months of observation

- analysis of clinical signs at various intervals during the observation period to predict probing attachment loss at 42 months compared with baseline

- clinical signs: dental plaque along the gingival margin, bleeding on probing, suppuration on probing, residual probing depth and increase in probing depth

- frequencies of the presence of supragingival plaque, bleeding and suppuration on probing calculated for each site from presence/absence scores available from examinations every third month (intervals: 3-12, 3-24, 3-36 and 3-42 months)
    - plaque and bleeding: percentage of positive scores of all examinations during the interval
    - suppuration: number of examinations with positive score

- attachment loss between 0-42 months determined from linear regression analysis of attachment level measurements performed every third month; threshold for loss: ≥ 1.5 mm; $P < 0.05$

- calculations of diagnostic predictability: percentage of sites with a given clinical sign that have undergone probing attachment loss

Results

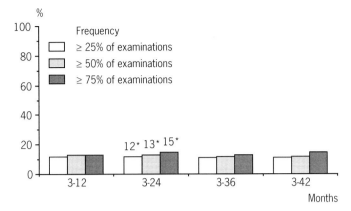

Fig. 4-19. Diagnostic predictability of plaque frequency scores.
*Interpretation: in the sites for which plaque was present ≥ 25% of the 8 examinations during 3-24 months, 12% demonstrated probing attachment loss during the 0- to 42-month time period; for presence ≥ 50% of the examinations, 13% lost attachment; for presence ≥ 75% of the examinations, 15% lost attachment

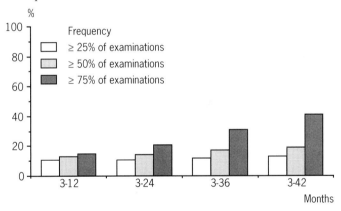

Fig. 4-20. Diagnostic predictability of bleeding frequency scores

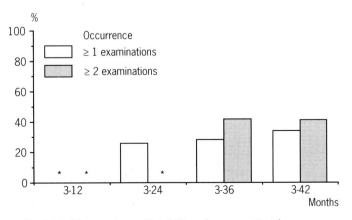

Fig. 4-21. Diagnostic predictability of suppuration frequency.
*Insufficient number of sites available for calculation

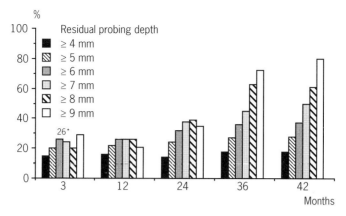

Fig. 4-22. Diagnostic predictability of residual probing depth.
*Interpretation: for the sites in which the residual probing depth was ≥ 6 mm at
3 months, 26% demonstrated probing attachment loss during the 0-42 months time
period

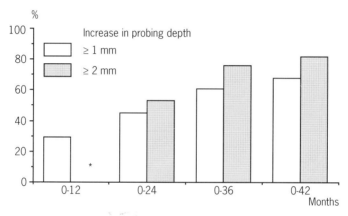

Fig. 4-23. Diagnostic predictability of increase in probing depth.
*Insufficient number of sites available for calculation

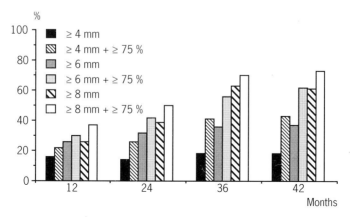

Fig. 4-24. Diagnostic predictability of residual probing depth (irrespective of bleeding on
probing) and residual probing depth plus bleeding frequency ≥ 75%

Comments

- The presence of dental plaque along the gingival margin at an increasing frequency of the examination intervals had but a limited effect on the chance of observing probing attachment loss between 0-42 months (Claffey et al.[29]) or 0-60 months (Badersten et al.[11]). In the Badersten et al. study, the presence of dental plaque at $\geq 75\%$ of the examination intervals during 5 years of observation reached a maximum predictive value of 30%. It is possible that the maintenance care, provided twice yearly in these studies, is a contributing factor to the limited effect of repeatedly observed plaque along the gingival margin.

- The relationship between bleeding on probing and probing attachment loss is illustrated by the increased predictive power associated with more frequently observed bleeding. In the Claffey et al. study, about 40% of the sites that bled at $\geq 75\%$ of the examinations between 3-42 months showed attachment loss during the 0- to 42-month period. Predictive values amounting to 20-40% for bleeding on probing have been observed in other studies as well (Badersten et al.[9,10], Lang et al.[58,59], Vanooteghem et al.[93], Chaves et al.[24]). Thus, bleeding on probing seems to have a moderate diagnostic value for prediction of continuous periodontal deterioration.

- Suppuration on probing was observed for a limited number of sites and was an infrequent occurrence for the sites in which it did take place. In the Claffey et al. study, the predictability value for suppuration occurring at 2-3 of the 14 examinations was similar to that found when a site showed bleeding on probing 11 times or more. Suppuration, therefore, when viewed in this light, may be a useful clinical sign.

- Increase in probing depth compared with baseline was strongly associated with probing attachment loss, particularly at later observation intervals. This indicates that deepening probing depths after treatment are most often explained by attachment loss and less often by coronal displacement of the gingival margin. For clinical purposes, the results mean that comparisons of recent probing depth measurements to baseline recordings should be recommended. The results may justify the concept that time-consuming probing attachment level measurements are not necessary in clinical practice, since probing depth change largely discloses the sites that have lost attachment.

- Residual probing depths 3-12 months after initial treatment showed limited predictability, including residual depths of ≥ 7 mm, ≥ 8 mm and ≥ 9 mm. This confirms the previous findings by Claffey et al.[28] (see pages 114-116). At later observation intervals the predictability of the deep residual depths increased significantly and amounted to 50-80%. As mentioned above, increased probing depth after initial treatment primarily seems to be a function of loss of probing attachment rather than an effect of gingival swelling. Therefore, the improved predictive power of residual probing depths at later observation intervals is related to the fact that the pools of deeper sites under analysis gradually will include more sites that have deepened plus lost probing attachment during the observation interval. For clinical purposes, these results indicate that a deep residual depth during the first year after treatment has a limited relationship with probing attachment loss. After a few years, however, the finding of a deep site probably indicates that the site has undergone attachment loss.

- Bleeding on probing at ≥ 75% of the examinations as an added requirement to residual probing depth improved the predictive power, particularly at later observation intervals. This provides support to the diagnostic value of bleeding on probing.

- In conclusion, the results confirm the use of the conventional recordings for monitoring purposes after periodontal treatment. However, longer observation intervals than those used traditionally for re-evaluation may be needed if the commonly used clinical signs are to reach meaningful diagnostic values.

GENERAL COMMENTS

- The finding that continuous attachment loss in untreated subjects is related to the baseline degree of periodontal involvement as expressed by probing depth, probing attachment level and periodontal bone level is not surprising. Subjects or individual sites with more baseline involvement than others have proven to be more susceptible. One would expect that these subjects or sites if left untreated would continue to show an increased risk of deterioration.

- Grbic & Lamster[40] (see pages 102-105) found an association between baseline degree of periodontal involvement and subsequent attachment loss in sites treated with scaling and root planing (without the use of local anesthesia). These observations are somewhat in contradiction to the findings of Badersten et al.[8,10] and Claffey et al.[29] presented in Chapter 3 (Effect of initial periodontal treatment). In the Badersten studies of nonmolar teeth, there was no indication that baseline deep probing depths or advanced bone loss was related to more probing attachment loss after treatment than less involved sites (pages 65-67). In the Claffey study, involving all teeth in the dentition, probing attachment loss ≥ 1.5 mm determined by regression analysis during 42 months after treatment was observed for 11% of sites initially ≤ 3.5 mm, for 7% of sites 4.0-6.5 and for 16% of sites initially ≥ 7 mm deep (see page 75).

- The limited association between plaque scores and continuous probing attachment loss in the studies reviewed may be related to the fact that the scores reflect the presence of supragingival plaque rather than subgingival plaque. Individuals with poor plaque control may be more or less prone to the development of subgingival plaque. The presence of subgingival plaque is more likely to be associated with disease progression than the presence of supragingival plaque. In addition, supragingival plaque scores only reflect differences in amounts of plaque. Differences in microbial composition of the plaque may be equally or more important relative to disease progression.

- The limited association of gingival redness to subsequent probing attachment loss may have several tentative explanations. An inflammatory involvement of the superficial gingival tissues may not correspond to inflamed conditions at the deeper and critical level: where the connective tissue fibers attach to the tooth. In addition, redness is a reflection of a vascular reaction, which need not necessarily be linked to the degradation of connective tissue.

- The rationale for the diagnostic use of bleeding on probing probably relates to its potential in reflecting inflammation close to the zone of connective tissue destruction. However, the limited association between bleeding on probing and subsequent attachment loss may be explained by the fact that probe penetration and vascular fragility may not be strongly linked to the factors responsible for collagen breakdown. In addition, the limitations of the presence/absence method of scoring used in the studies need to be considered. These limitations were elucidated in Chapter 2 (Methods of examination) (see pages 16-25, 28-29, 57).

- The difficulties in predicting the short- and long-term outcome of initial periodontal therapy at a site level were highlighted by the findings of Claffey et al.[28], Badersten et al.[11] and Claffey et al.[29] (see pages 114-124). Apparently, no clinical characteristic adequately predicts continuous deterioration. The fact that increase in probing depth after treatment showed a close relationship to probing attachment loss is of importance for evaluation purposes, since probing depth measurements may substitute for the more cumbersome probing attachment level measurements. However, the probing depth changes can be considered to be an after-the-fact reflection of probing attachment loss and therefore not truly predictive.

- Conceivably, an experienced clinician could have accumulated some feel for the conditions often leading to clinical failure, conditions that could not be identified by a more objective and systematic approach to the analysis. However, the results of the study by Vanooteghem et al.[94] indicate that the predictability of the subjective judgments of experienced clinicians may also be limited (see pages 112-113).

- The studies on the diagnostic value of the various clinical signs have been performed using pools of sites and groups of patients. Thus, the analyses have been based on the assumption that all sites and all patients should show a similar response to a given sign. This may or may not be true. In fact, the modest predictive results in the studies can be interpreted to indicate that this is generally not true. A given sign could be closely linked to disease activity in one patient but not in another patient. Such variations may also exist from one site to another within the same individual.

- The inflammatory response of the living body is basically a protective mechanism but includes destructive components also. The balance of these 2 aspects and their role in periodontal disease is not known. Therefore, it should come as no surprise that comparatively crude parameters of gingival inflammation show limited association with disease progression. More specific indicators may be needed, such as identification of the microorganisms actually causing the disease or identification of products in the gingival fluid associated with ongoing disease activity and tissue destruction.

CHAPTER 5

Case reports – re-evaluation status

The purpose of this chapter is to provide some examples of teeth and surfaces with a questionable clinical status at 3-month re-evaluation following initial periodontal therapy and to present the subsequent events for these sites.

The sites were selected from the 17 patients participating in the study by Claffey et al.[29]. The treatment, maintenance care and overall results of treatment in these patients are described on pages 70-77.

The selection of cases to be presented in a context such as this needs to be judicious to avoid presentation of nonrepresentative examples. The following approach was used:

- Selection was limited to approximal surfaces, since periodontal problems are more common for these surfaces than for buccal and lingual.

- Both sites from each selected approximal tooth surface had a probing depth ≥ 6 mm and showed bleeding on probing at 3-month re-evaluation. Thus, for selected distal surfaces, both the distobuccal and distolingual sites complied with these criteria. For selected mesial surfaces, both mesiobuccal and mesiolingual sites complied. The fulfillment of these requirements for both sites of the approximal surface, as opposed to a single site, should have increased the likelihood of selection of areas with potential problems.

- All of the identified cases are presented.

In the 17 patients, there were 338 teeth and 676 approximal surfaces. The selection process resulted in the identification of 11 approximal surfaces meeting the criteria (6 distal and 5 mesial). Nine patients had 1 such surface each and 1 patient had 2 surfaces. Case details relating to the 11 surfaces are presented on pages 133-176.

Brief, general information is given for each of the 10 patients. Plaque scores, bleeding scores and the percentage of probing depths ≥ 6 mm for the entire dentition are presented for each patient throughout the 42-month observation interval. In addition, recordings at 0, 3 and 42 months for all sites of the tooth in question are shown. Also included is a set of pretreatment radiographs of the entire dentition, together with pre- and posttreatment radiographs (if available) of the area of interest.

Data from all examinations between 0-42 months are presented for the selected approximal surfaces. Probing depths and probing attachment levels are presented using a graphic display, thus facilitating a longitudinal evaluation of the recordings.

The international tooth numbering system is used. However, the first time a tooth is mentioned, the corresponding United States system number is placed within brackets: 41 (25), 42 (26), etc.

Recordings are presented at 6 sites for nonmolar teeth; 8 sites for maxillary molars; and 10 sites for mandibular molars as demonstrated below (abbreviations explained on the following page):

Table 5-1

Sites recorded for nonmolar teeth, maxillary molars and mandibular molars

Nonmolar teeth

MB		B		DB
ML		L		DL

Maxillary molars

MB	MBM	BF	MBD	DB
MF		L		DF

Mandibular molars

MB	MBM	BF	MBD	DB
ML	MLM	LF	MLD	DL

MB:	mesiobuccal	MBM:	mid-buccal of mesial root
ML:	mesiolingual	MLM:	mid-lingual of mesial root
MF:	mesial furcation		

B:	buccal	MBD:	mid-buccal of distal root
BF:	buccal furcation	MLD:	mid-lingual of distal root
L:	lingual		
LF:	lingual furcation		

DB:	distobuccal
DL:	distolingual
DF:	distal furcation

An example of the graphs used to present the longitudinal events for the selected sites is given below:

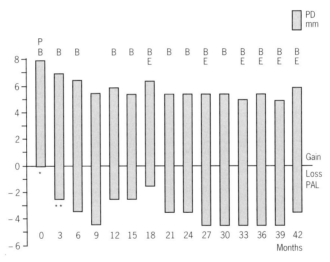

Fig. 5-1. CN, tooth 14, distobuccal. Display of scores for probing depth (PD), probing attachment level (PAL), plaque (P), bleeding (B) and exudate/suppuration on probing (E) throughout 42 months of observation.

Interpretation

*   At 0 months, the distobuccal site showed a probing depth (PD) of 8 mm, bleeding on probing (B) and plaque (P). The probing attachment level (PAL, base of probeable pocket) at 0 months provides the 0-axis for orientation of subsequent (3-42 months) probing measurements.

** At 3 months, the site showed 2.5 mm loss of probing attachment (the base of the bar now being located 2.5 mm below the 0-month level). The gingival recession amounted to 1.0 mm (the top of the

3-month bar located 1.0 mm below the top level of the 0-month bar). The probing depth had increased from 8.0 mm to 9.5 mm (total heights of bars). Overall, during the 42-month period, this site remained 9-10 mm deep, lost 4-5 mm of probing attachment and exhibited bleeding (B) and exudate/suppuration on probing (E).

CASE C.N.

Age:	40 years
Sex:	Male
Number of remaining teeth:	23
Selected tooth and surface:	14 (5) distal
Medical history:	None relevant
Medication:	None
Smoker:	Yes, 1 pack/day
Dental history:	Irregular dental treatment
	No previous periodontal therapy
	Maxillary incisors lost
	due to periodontal disease

Clinical findings, entire dentition

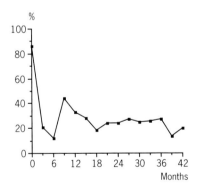

Fig. 5-2. Plaque scores (%)

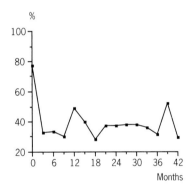

Fig. 5-3. Bleeding scores (%)

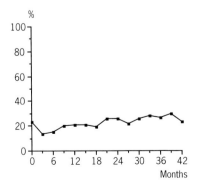

Fig. 5-4. Probing depths ≥ 6 mm (%)

Radiographs, entire dentition

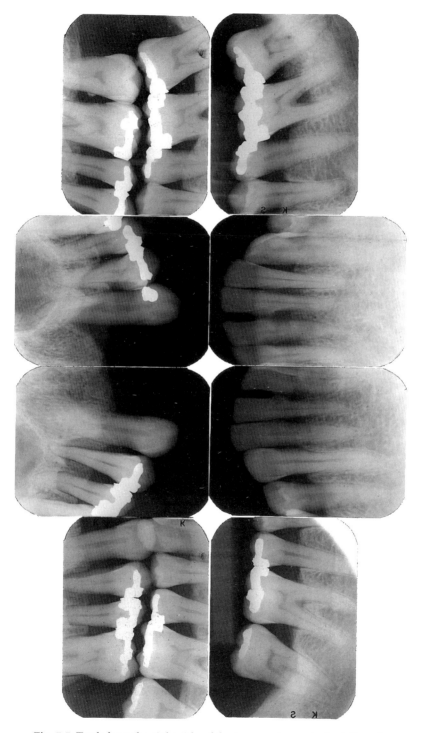

Fig. 5-5. Teeth from the right side of the jaw are shown to the left, and teeth from the left side to the right.

Clinical findings, tooth 14

Table 5-2
Probing depth in mm, presence of plaque (P), bleeding (B) and exudate/suppuration on probing (E) for the examined sites at initial, 3-month and 42-month examinations

Initial

DB*	B	MB
8.0^{PB}	2.0	3.0^{PB}
7.0^{PB}	6.0	6.0^{PB}
DL*	L	ML

3 months

DB*	B	MB
9.5^{B}	2.0	3.0^{B}
6.5^{B}	5.0	6.0^{B}
DL*	L	ML

42 months

DB*	B	MB
9.5^{BE}	2.0	4.5^{B}
10.0^{P}	5.0	7.0^{B}
DL*	L	ML

*Selected approximal surfaces indicated in bold

Radiographs, tooth 14

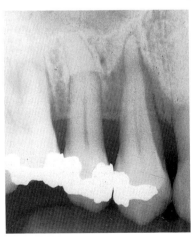

Fig. 5-6. Initial

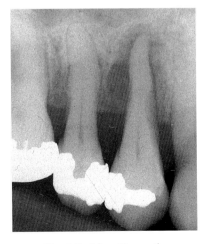

Fig. 5-7. After 42 months

Clinical findings, 14 distal

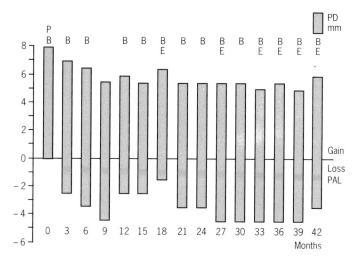

Fig. 5-8. CN, tooth 14, distobuccal

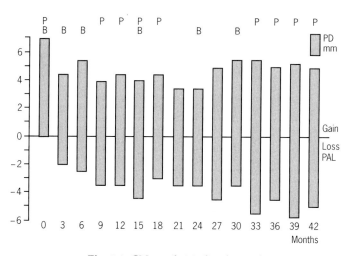

Fig. 5-9. CN, tooth 14, distolingual

Comments

- Overall, the plaque and bleeding scores improved after therapy; the percentage of probing depths ≥ 6 mm did not.

- Before treatment, the lesion at the distal surface approached the root apex and extended over the palatal to the mesial surface.

- Persistence of bleeding and a high frequency of suppuration was seen for the distobuccal aspect. Both sites increased in probing depth and lost probing attachment. At 42 months, the lesion had extended periapically.

CASE E.L.

Age:	37 years
Sex:	Male
Number of remaining teeth:	28
Selected tooth and surface:	26 (14) distal
Medical history:	None relevant
Medication:	None
Smoker:	No
Dental history:	Irregular dental treatment
	No previous periodontal therapy

Clinical findings, entire dentition

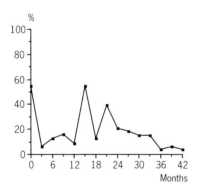

Fig. 5-10. Plaque scores (%)

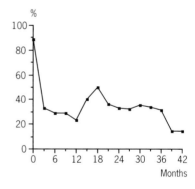

Fig. 5-11. Bleeding scores (%)

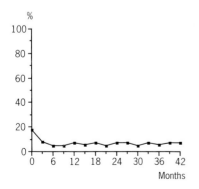

Fig. 5-12. Probing depths ≥ 6 mm (%)

Radiographs, entire dentition

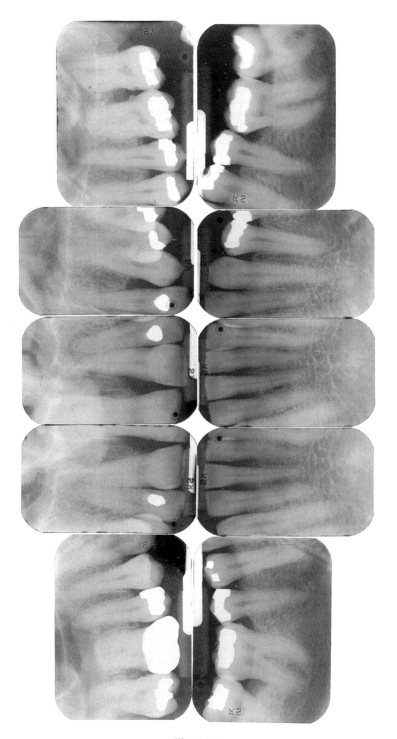

Fig. 5-13

Clinical findings, tooth 26

Table 5-3

Initial

	MB	MBM	BF	MBD	**DB**
	5.5^B	2.0^B	6.5^B	6.5^B	10.0^B
	4.5^{PB}		2.0^B		8.5^{PB}
	MF		L		**DF**

3 months

	MB	MBM	BF	MBD	**DB**
	3.5^B	1.5	4.0	4.5	9.0^B
	3.0		2.0		9.0^B
	MF		L		**DF**

42 months

	MB	MBM	BF	MBD	**DB**
	3.0	2.0	4.0	4.0^B	10.5^B
	3.0		2.0		15.0^B
	MF		L		**DF**

Radiographs, tooth 26

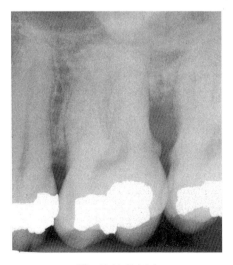
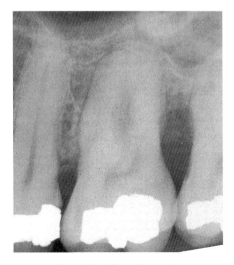

Fig. 5-14. Initial   **Fig. 5-15**. After 52 months

Clinical findings, 26 distal

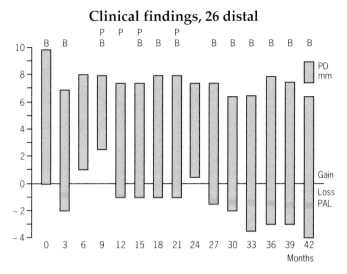

Fig. 5-16. EL, tooth 26, distobuccal

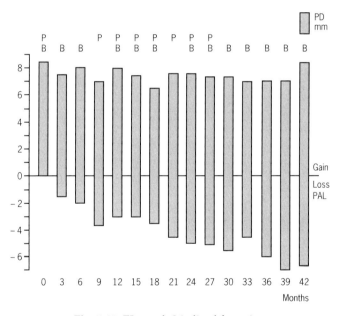

Fig. 5-17. EL, tooth 26, distal furcation

Comments

- This 37-year-old patient had localized areas of severe disease. Before treatment, tooth 26 had furcation involvement distally. At 3 months, no improvement could be seen for this surface.

- The distal lesion deepened, particularly at the furcation, showed loss of attachment and bled persistently during the 42-month period. Deterioration could also be seen radiographically.

CASE I.E.

Age:	62 years
Sex:	Female
Number of remaining teeth:	24 (excluding wisdom teeth and 2 teeth extracted before treatment)
Selected tooth and surface:	37 (18) mesial
Medical history:	None relevant
Medication:	None
Smoker:	Yes, 1 pack/day
Dental history:	Irregular dental treatment No previous periodontal therapy 1 maxillary and 1 mandibular incisor lost due to periodontitis

Clinical findings, entire dentition

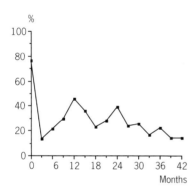

Fig. 5-18. Plaque scores (%)

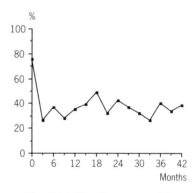

Fig. 5-19. Bleeding scores (%)

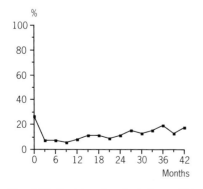

Fig. 5-20. Probing depths ≥ 6 mm (%)

Radiographs, entire dentition

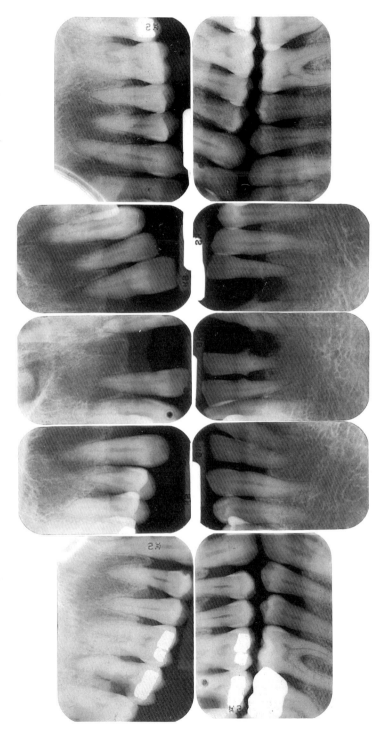

Fig. 5-21

Clinical findings, tooth 37

Table 5-4

Initial

	MB	MBM	BF	MBD	DB
	6.0^{PB}	6.5^{PB}	7.0^{PB}	-*	7.0^{PB}
	9.0^{PB}	5.0^{PB}	-	-	5.5^{PB}
	ML	MLM	LF	MLD	DL

3 months

	MB	MBM	BF	MBD	DB
	6.5^{PB}	3.5^{P}	4.0^{PB}	-	4.0
	8.0^{PB}	2.0	-	-	5.0
	ML	MLM	LF	MLD	DL

42 months

	MB	MBM	BF	MBD	DB
	7.0	7.0	4.0	-	5.0^{PB}
	8.0	3.0	-	-	7.0^{B}
	ML	MLM	LF	MLD	DL

* Recordings not available

Radiographs, tooth 37

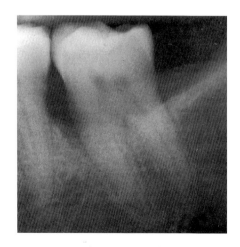

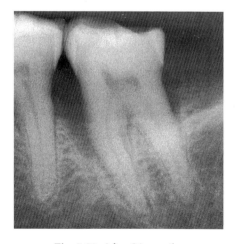

Fig. 5-22. Initial

Fig. 5-23. After 84 months

Clinical findings, 37 mesial

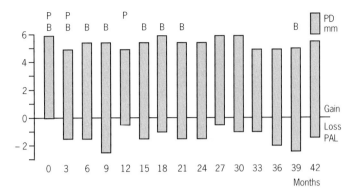

Fig. 5-24. IE, tooth 37, mesiobuccal

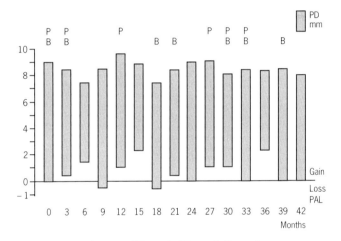

Fig. 5-25. IE, tooth 37, mesiolingual

Comments

- This patient had localized posterior lesions but showed most bone loss in maxillary and mandibular incisor areas. Before treatment, 17 (2) and 41 (25) were extracted. An intraosseous lesion was seen at the mesial surface of tooth 37.

- The probing measurements during the 42-month period possibly indicate some deterioration for the mesiobuccal but not for the mesiolingual site. The loss of attachment for the mesiobuccal site, however, could conceivably have been inflicted during instrumentation. The radiograph taken after 7 years did not disclose any deterioration. The variations of probing recordings during the 42 months are probably related to measurement errors, such as differences in placement of the probe at the site for measurement.

CASE J.O.

Age:	43 years
Sex:	Male
Number of remaining teeth:	27 (excluding wisdom teeth)
Selected tooth and surface:	27 (15) distal
Medical history:	Hypertension, hepatitis A 10 years before
Medication:	Clonidine hydrochloride and chlorthalidone
Smoker:	No
Dental history:	Regular dental treatment Received periodontal therapy in the past without success

Clinical findings, entire dentition

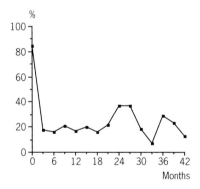

Fig. 5-26. Plaque scores (%)

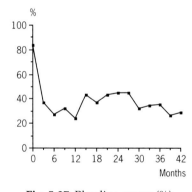

Fig. 5-27. Bleeding scores (%)

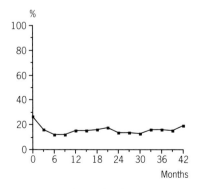

Fig. 5-28. Probing depths ≥ 6 mm (%)

145

Radiographs, entire dentition

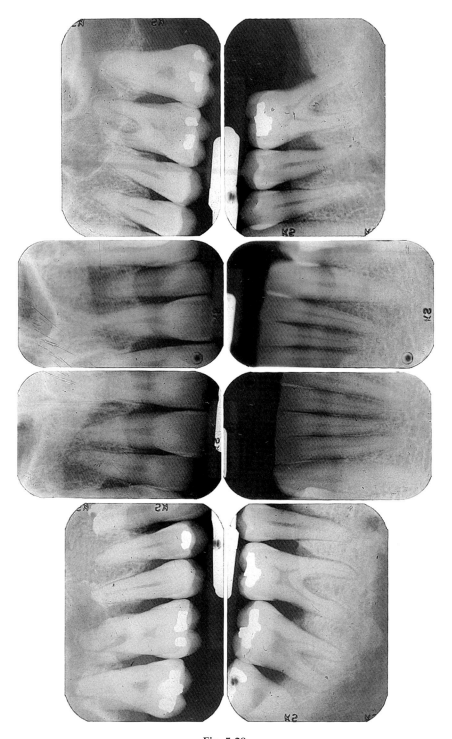

Fig. 5-29

Clinical findings, tooth 27

Table 5-5

Initial

	MB	MBM	BF	MBD	**DB**
	5.0^{PB}	2.5^{PB}	3.0^{PB}	3.0^{PB}	8.0^{PB}
	5.5^{PB}		5.0^{PB}		8.5^{PB}
	MF		L		**DF***

3 months

	MB	MBM	BF	MBD	**DB**
	3.5^P	2.0 B	3.0^B	4.0^P	6.5^B
	4.5^{PB}		4.0		7.0^{PB}
	MF		L		**DF***

42 months

	MB	MBM	BF	MBD	**DB**
	5.0^{PB}	2.0	2.5	3.0^P	8.0^{PB}
	3.5^{PB}		3.0		8.0^{PB}
	MF		L		**DF***

* This tooth had fused roots without genuine furcations

Radiographs, tooth 27

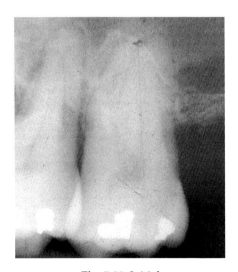
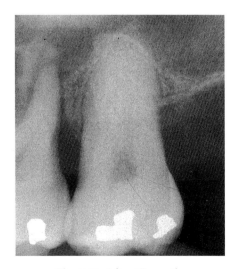

Fig. 5-30. Initial   **Fig. 5-31**. After 67 months

Clinical findings, 27 distal

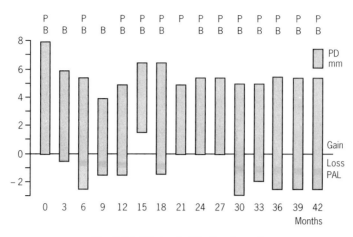

Fig. 5-32. JO, tooth 27, distobuccal

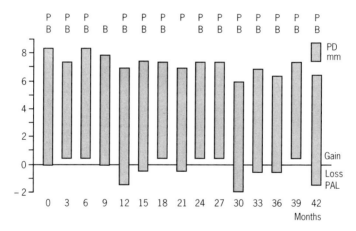

Fig. 5-33. JO, tooth 27, distolingual

Comments

- This 43-year-old male had a history of unsuccessful periodontal treatment and a number of intraosseous lesions throughout the dentition.

- Tooth 27 had marked bone loss and deep probing depths at the distal surface. At 3 months, there was little improvement in probing depth and bleeding at this location, possibly related to the soft tissue anatomy in this region.

- Loss of attachment probably occurred for the distobuccal site over the 42 months. Note persistent bleeding on probing for both sites. Radiographically, no change could be observed after 67 months.

CASE J.S.

Age:	40 years
Sex:	Male
Number of remaining teeth:	24
Selected tooth and surface:	14 (5) distal
Medical history:	None relevant
Medication:	None
Smoker:	No
Dental history:	Irregular dental treatment
	No previous periodontal treatment
	Several molars lost due to periodontal disease

Clinical findings, entire dentition

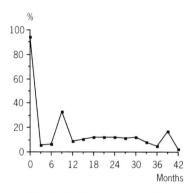

Fig. 5-34. Plaque scores (%)

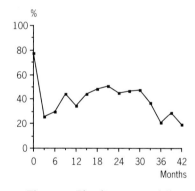

Fig. 5-35. Bleeding scores (%)

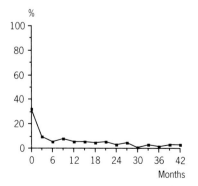

Fig. 5-36. Probing depths ≥ 6 mm (%)

Radiographs, entire dentition

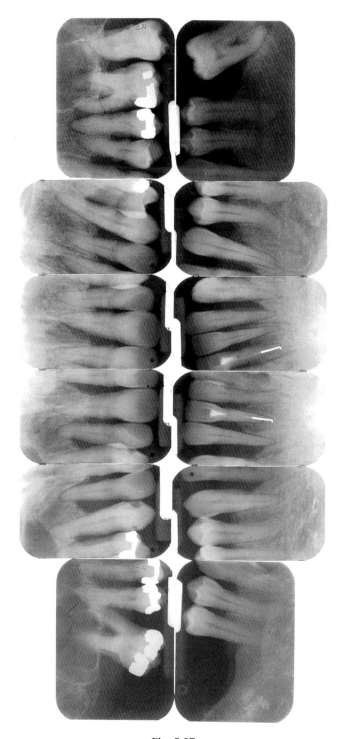

Fig. 5-37

Clinical findings, tooth 14

Table 5-6

Initial

DB	B	MB
10.0^{PBE}	2.0^B	5.5^{PB}
7.5^{PB}	6.5^{PB}	6.0^{PB}
DL	L	ML

3 months

DB	B	MB
7.5^B	2.0^B	2.5
8.5^B	4.5	3.5
DL	L	ML

42 months

DB	B	MB
3.0^B	1.5	2.5
6.0	3.0	3.0
DL	L	ML

Radiographs, tooth 14

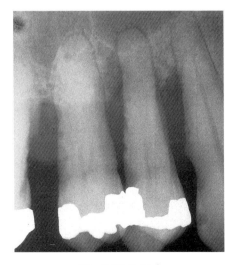
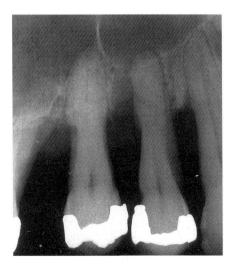

Fig. 5-38. Initial   Fig. 5-39. After 24 months

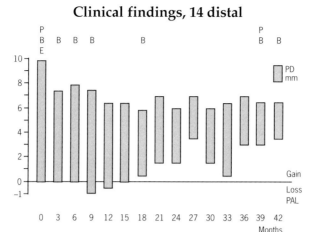

Fig. 5-40. JS, tooth 14, distobuccal

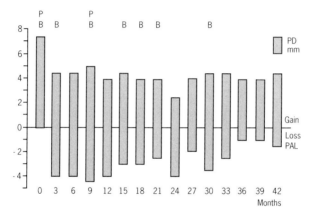

Fig. 5-41. JS, tooth 14, distolingual

Comments

- In spite of the advanced bone loss, this 40-year-old patient had limited tooth mobility. All available teeth were treated. Plaque scores and the percentage of probing depths ≥ 6 mm improved dramatically.

- Tooth 14 had marked bone loss initially. Distally, this loss extended close to the root apex. Three months after treatment the status for this surface was still questionable.

- The distobuccal measurements showed continuous improvement during the 42-month interval. The distolingual loss of attachment seen at 3 months could possibly be explained by trauma from instrumentation during initial treatment.

- Radiographically, no change was observed after 24 months.

CASE K.F.

Age:	61 years
Sex:	Female
Number of remaining teeth:	22
Selected tooth and surface:	17 (2) mesial
Medical history:	Glaucoma
Medication:	Pilocarpine
Smoker:	Yes, one half pack/day
Dental history:	Regular dental treatment
	No previous periodontal therapy

Clinical findings, entire dentition

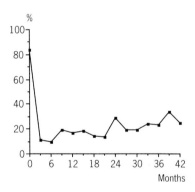

Fig. 5-42. Plaque scores (%)

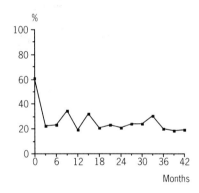

Fig. 5-43. Bleeding scores (%)

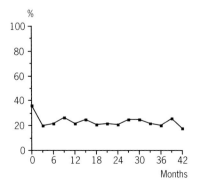

Fig. 5-44. Probing depths ≥ 6 mm (%)

Radiographs, entire dentition

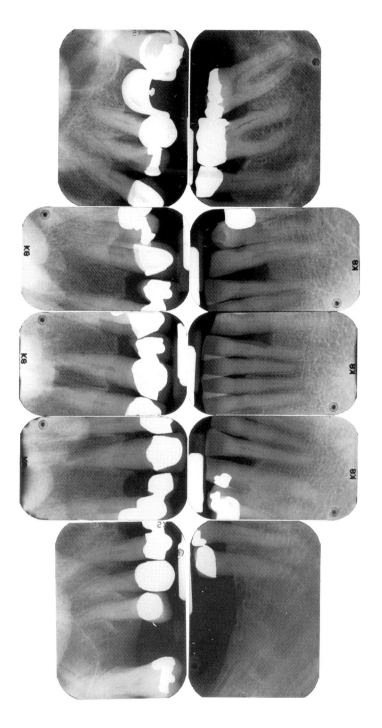

Fig. 5-45

Clinical findings, tooth 17

Table 5-7

Initial

	DB	MBD	BF	MBM	**MB**
	8.0^{PB}		3.0^{P}	2.0^{P}	7.0^{PB}
	8.0^{PB}		4.5^{P}		7.0^{PB}
	DF		L		**MF**

3 months

	DB	MBD	BF	MBM	**MB**
	7.0^{P}		3.0	2.0	6.0^{PB}
	9.0^{P}		3.5		6.0^{PB}
	DF		L		**MF**

42 months

	DB	MBD	BF	MBM	**MB**
	3.0		3.0	2.0	3.0^{P}
	6.5		4.0		9.0^{PB}
	DF		L		**MF**

Radiographs, tooth 17

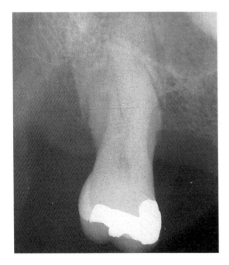

Fig. 5-46. Initial

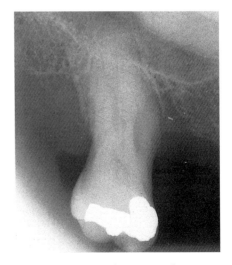

Fig. 5-47. After 29 months

Clinical findings, 17 mesial

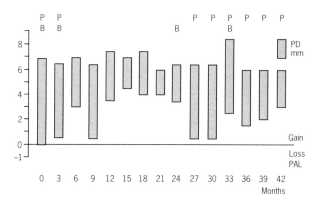

Fig. 5-48. KF, tooth 17, mesiobuccal

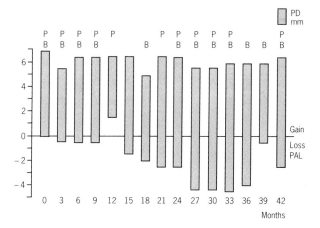

Fig. 5-49. KF, tooth 17, mesial furcation

Comments

- This patient showed bone loss throughout the dentition and a high percentage of probing depths ≥ 6 mm before treatment.

- Tooth 17 had deep pockets and furcation involvement both mesially and distally.

- The mesiobuccal probing measurements indicated improvement during the observation interval. The mesial furcation site gradually lost attachment between 15 and 27 months. The reversal in attachment levels for this site at the end of the observation interval could be an effect of probing error or possibly a reflection of improved tissue tonus.

- Radiographically, no change could be seen after 29 months.

CASE L.S.

Age:	50 years
Sex:	Male
Number of remaining teeth:	16 (excluding 2 teeth extracted before treatment)
Selected tooth and surface:	37 (18) distal
Medical history:	None relevant
Medication:	None
Smoker:	Yes, 1 pack/day
Dental history:	Sporadic dental treatment No previous periodontal treatment Anterior teeth lost due to caries

Clinical findings, entire dentition

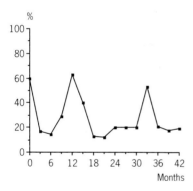

Fig. 5-50. Plaque scores (%)

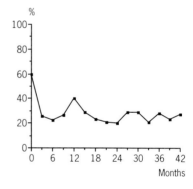

Fig. 5-51. Bleeding scores (%)

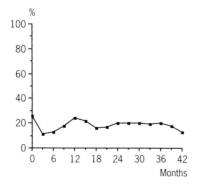

Fig. 5-52. Probing depths ≥ 6 mm (%)

Radiographs, entire dentition

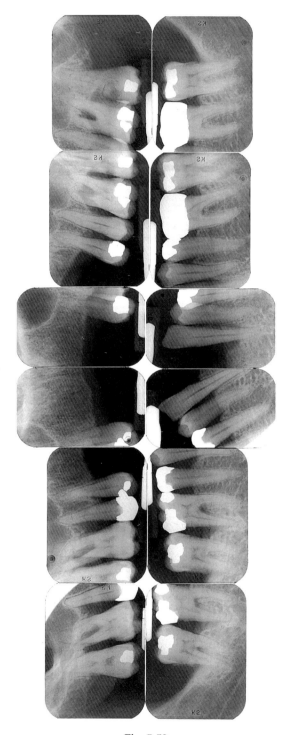

Fig. 5-53

Clinical findings, tooth 37

Table 5-8

Initial

	MB	MBM	BF	MBD	**DB**
	4.0^{PB}	3.0^P	5.0^P	-*	7.5^{PB}
	6.0^B	2.0^P	6.0^P	-	10.5^{PB}
	ML	MLM	LF	MLD	**DL**

3 months

	MB	MBM	BF	MBD	**DB**
	3.0	3.0^P	6.5	-	9.0^{PB}
	5.0^P	3.0^P	6.0^{PB}	-	13.0^{PB}
	ML	MLM	LF	MLD	**DL**

42 months

	MB	MBM	BF	MBD	**DB**
	4.0	3.0	5.5^B	-	8.0^P
	7.0^P	2.0	9.0^{PB}	-	9.0^P
	ML	MLM	LF	MLD	**DL**

* Recordings not available

Radiographs, tooth 37

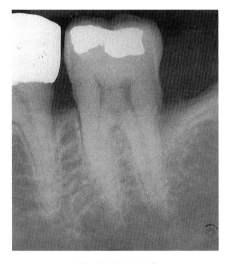 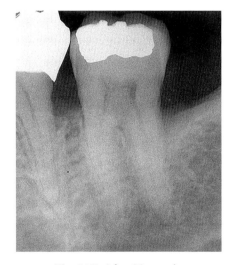

Fig. 5-54. Initial   **Fig. 5-55**. After 33 months

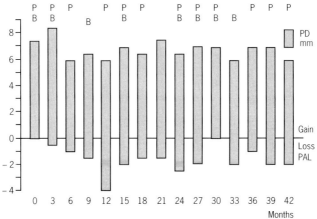

Fig. 5-56. LS, tooth 37, distobuccal

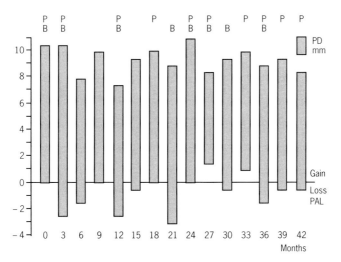

Fig. 5-57. LS, tooth 37, distolingual

Comments

- Before treatment, 16 (3) and 27 (15) were extracted.

- Tooth 37 showed a vertical defect and deep probing depths at the distal surface. At 3 months, no improvement was seen for this surface.

- The probing measurements during the 42 months of observation may possibly indicate some loss of attachment for the distobuccal site but not for the distolingual site. The radiograph taken after 33 months did not disclose any deterioration.

CASE M.B.

Age:	43 years
Sex:	Female
Number of remaining teeth:	18
Selected tooth and surface:	21 (9) mesial
Medical history:	None relevant
Medication:	None
Smoker:	No
Dental history:	Regular dental treatment No previous periodontal therapy

Clinical findings, entire dentition

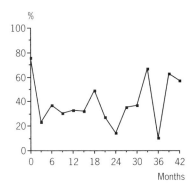

Fig. 5-58. Plaque scores (%)

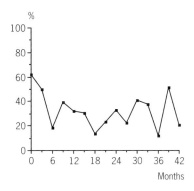

Fig. 5-59. Bleeding scores (%)

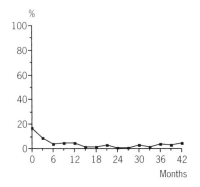

Fig. 5-60. Probing depths ≥ 6 mm (%)

Radiographs, entire dentition

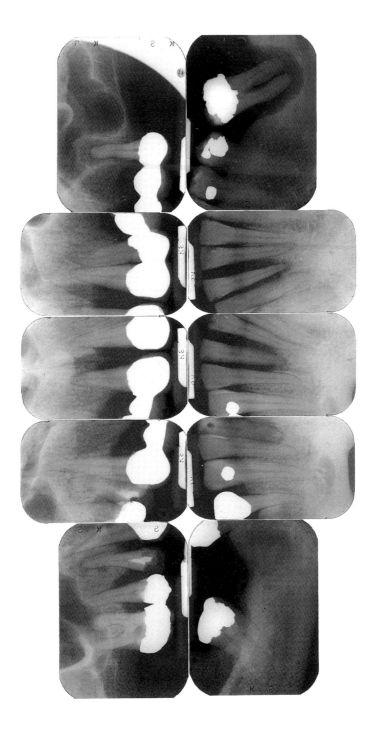

Fig. 5-61

Clinical findings, tooth 21

Table 5-9

Initial

MB	B	DB
11.0^{PB}	7.0^{PB}	4.5^{P}
11.0^{PB}	10.5^{PB}	3.5^{PB}
ML	L	DL

3 months

MB	B	DB
8.0^{PBE}	5.0^{P}	4.0^{B}
8.5^{PB}	8.5^{PB}	6.0^{B}
ML	L	DL

42 months

MB	B	DB
4.0^{PB}	2.0^{P}	2.0^{P}
6.0^{P}	3.5^{P}	2.0^{P}
ML	L	DL

Radiographs, tooth 21

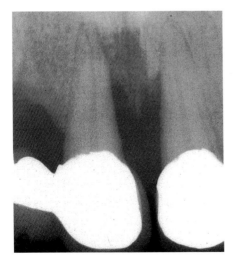 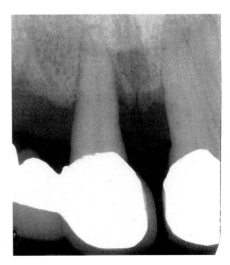

Fig. 5-62. Initial   **Fig. 5-63**. After 92 months

Clinical findings, 21 mesial

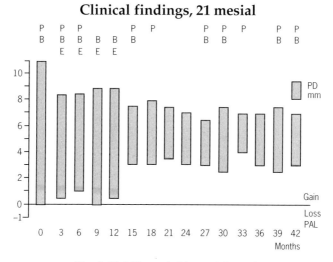

Fig. 5-64. MB, tooth 21, mesiobuccal

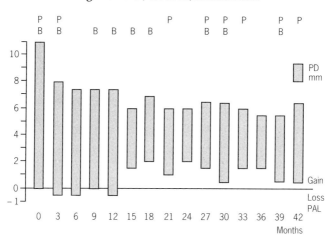

Fig. 5-65. MB, tooth 21, mesiolingual

Comments

- This 43-year-old woman had not received adequate treatment for her dental problems. Tooth 37 (18) was extracted. Tooth 41 (25) was treated and responded well.

- The mesial surface of 21 showed a deep intraosseous lesion extending over the buccal and lingual surfaces.

- Although probing depths decreased somewhat, the mesial surface showed suppuration and bleeding at 3 months. However, marked improvement occurred at 15 months (possibly due to maintenance treatment) and was sustained over the 42-month observation interval. Radiographically, no change could be seen after 92 months.

CASE M.H.

Age:	47 years
Sex:	Female

Number of remaining teeth: 23

Selected teeth and surfaces: 24 (12) mesial
46 (30) mesial

Medical history: Hypothyroid, anemic periodically

Medication: Benztropine mesylate,
trifluoperazine, levothyroxine sodium

Smoker: No

Dental history: Irregular dental treatment
No previous periodontal treatment

Clinical findings, entire dentition

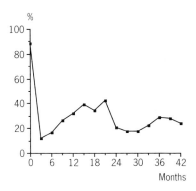

Fig. 5-66. Plaque scores (%)

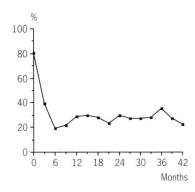

Fig. 5-67. Bleeding scores (%)

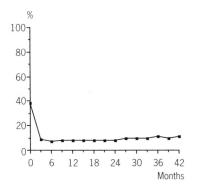

Fig. 5-68. Probing depths ≥ 6 mm (%)

Radiographs, entire dentition

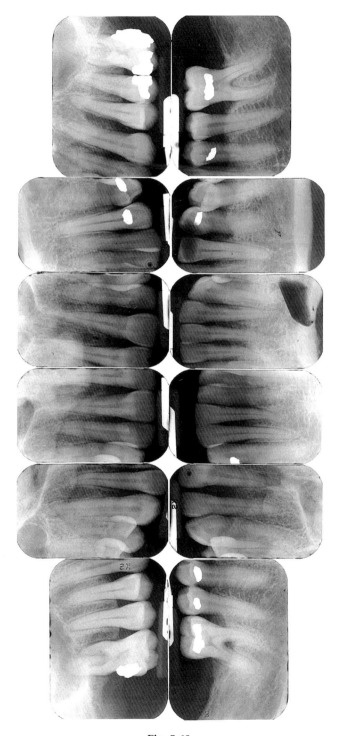

Fig. 5-69

Clinical findings, tooth 24

Table 5-10

Initial

MB	B	DB
10.5^{PB}	7.0	7.0^{PB}
10.0^{PB}	7.0^{PB}	6.0^{PB}
ML	L	DL

3 months

MB	B	DB
8.5^{B}	6.0^{B}	4.0^{PB}
7.5^{B}	6.5^{B}	4.0^{B}
ML	L	DL

42 months

MB	B	DB
7.0^{PB}	6.0^{B}	9.0^{BE}
9.0^{B}	8.0^{B}	8.0^{PB}
ML	L	DL

Radiographs, tooth 24

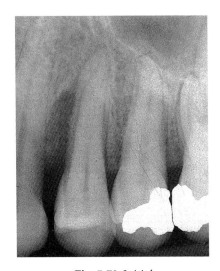 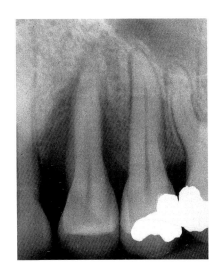

Fig. 5-70. Initial   Fig. 5-71. After 34 months

Clinical findings, 24 mesial

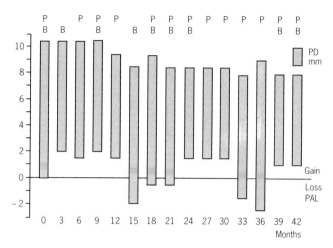

Fig. 5-72. MH, tooth 24, mesiobuccal

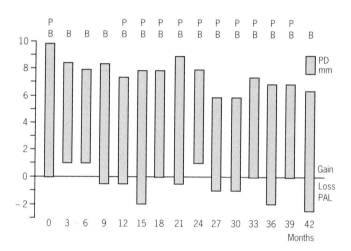

Fig. 5-73. MH, tooth 24, mesiolingual

Comments

- The percentage of depths ≥ 6 mm was reduced notably after treatment.

- Tooth 26 demonstrated a deep, mesial intraosseous lesion with furcation involvement.

- Little change was observed for the mesial surface during the 42 months. However, the distal surface - after initial improvement - deteriorated subsequently (perhaps indicating an extension from the mesial surface through the furcation area). Deterioration was radiographically evident at 34 months.

Clinical findings, tooth 46

Table 5-11

Initial

	DB	MBD	BF	MBM	**MB**
	6.0^{PB}	-*	8.0^B	2.0^B	7.5^{PB}
	6.0^{PB}	-	7.5^{PB}	4.0^{PB}	8.0^{PB}
	DL	MLD	LF	MLM	**ML**

3 months

	DB	MBD	BF	MBM	**MB**
	3.0	-	7.0^B	2.0	6.5^B
	5.0	-	6.0^B	5.0	6.5^B
	DL	MLD	LF	MLM	**ML**

42 months

	DB	MBD	BF	MBM	**MB**
	2.5^P	-	7.0^{BE}	2.0	6.5^B
	4.0^P	-	4.5	2.0	6.0^B
	DL	MLD	LF	MLM	**ML**

* Recordings not available

Radiographs, tooth 46

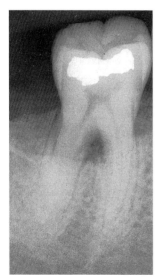 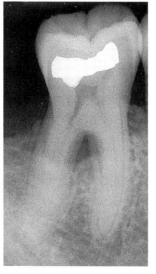 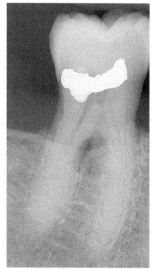

Fig. 5-74. Initial   **Fig. 5-75**. After 34 months   **Fig. 5-76**. After 64 months

Clinical findings, 46 mesial

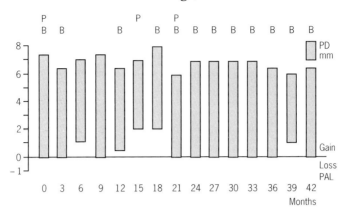

Fig. 5-77. MH, tooth 46, mesiobuccal

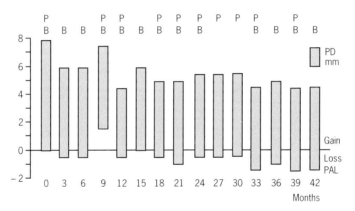

Fig. 5-78. MH, tooth 46, mesiolingual

Comments

- Tooth 46 had buccal furcation involvement but limited approximal bone loss.

- The mesial sites, questionable at 3 months, showed little change during the 42 months of observation. Bleeding occurred at most of the recordings.

- The buccal furcation lesion showed suppuration at 42 months. However, the probing depth for this site at 42 months and the available radiographs after 34 and 64 months did not suggest deterioration.

CASE P.J.

Age:	60 years
Sex:	Male
Number of remaining teeth:	24
Selected tooth and surface:	37 (18) distal
Medical history:	Heart attack 6 months previously
Medication:	Nitroglycerin
Smoker:	No
Dental history:	Irregular dental treatment
	No previous periodontal therapy

Clinical findings, entire dentition

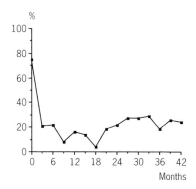

Fig. 5-79. Plaque scores (%)

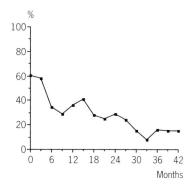

Fig. 5-80. Bleeding scores (%)

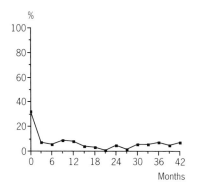

Fig. 5-81. Probing depths ≥ 6 mm (%)

Radiographs, entire dentition

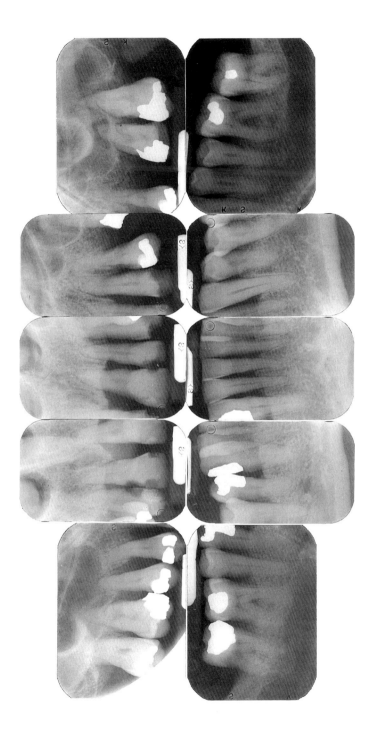

Fig. 5-82

Clinical findings, tooth 37

Table 5-12

Initial

MB	MBM	BF	MBD	**DB**
6.0^P	2.5^B	3.0^B	4.0^B	7.5^{PB}
4.5^{PB}	4.0^{PB}	5.5^{PB}	6.0^{PB}	6.5^{PB}
ML	MLM	LF	MLD	**DL**

3 months

MB	MBM	BF	MBD	**DB**
4.0^B	2.0^P	3.0^P	3.0^P	6.5^{PB}
3.0^{PB}	3.0^B	5.0^P	4.5^P	8.0^{PB}
ML	MLM	LF	MLD	**DL**

42 months

MB	MBM	BF	MBD	**DB**
4.0	2.0	2.0	2.0	4.0^P
3.5^B	2.5	3.0^P	3.5^P	5.0^P
ML	MLM	LF	MLD	**DL**

Radiograph, tooth 37

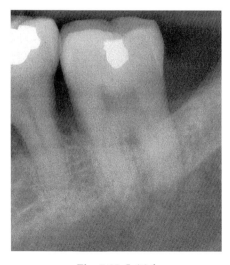

Fig. 5-83. Initial

Clinical findings, 37 distal

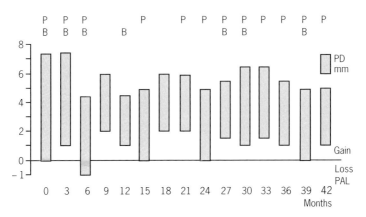

Fig. 5-84. PJ, tooth 37, distobuccal

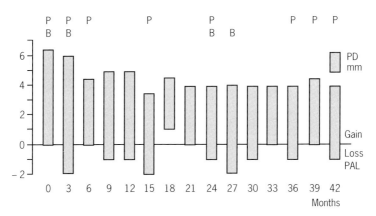

Fig. 5-85. PJ, tooth 37, distolingual

Comments

- This patient had marked bone loss throughout the dentition. Teeth 26 (14) and 27 (15) were extracted prior to treatment.

- Tooth 37 appears to have an intraosseous lesion at the distal surface. Both sites showed questionable status at 3 months but improved thereafter.

- Fluctuations in probing depths at this site may reflect difficulties with access during probing.

GENERAL COMMENTS

- The cases presented in this chapter generally showed advanced period-ontitis. Treatment resulted in improved plaque and bleeding scores and a reduced percentage of probing depths ≥ 6 mm. The degree of improvement varied among the patients. Plaque and bleeding scores often showed noticeable variability within individual subjects during the 42-month observation interval.

- A more complete presentation of the individual outcome of treatment for the entire dentition may have been desirable. However, the scope of this chapter was limited to re-evaluation issues on a tooth surface basis. General information on the patient was included to provide some background for the site evaluations.

- In the studies by Badersten et al.[11] and Claffey et al.[29], the diagnostic predictability of clinical signs for subsequent probing attachment loss in individual sites was found to be limited (see pages 117-124). For the case reports presented in this chapter, it was decided that both of the examined sites for an approximal surface should have a questionable 3-month re-evaluation status. This was done to increase the likelihood of selecting areas with potential problems. A review of the cases indicates that about one half of the selected approximal surfaces showed subsequent probing attachment loss allied to frequent bleeding at 1 or both of the sites - features suggesting an ongoing disease process. The predictability at 3-month re-evaluation for subsequent probing attachment loss at either site of an approximal surface may be somewhat enhanced compared with that seen when similar criteria were applied to individual sites by Badersten et al.[11] and Claffey et al.[29]. However, as only 11 approximal surfaces were reviewed, this material may not be representative.

- Other factors than residual probing depth and bleeding on probing may be more important relative to subsequent deterioration. Interestingly, all of the selected lesions that showed unquestionable loss of attachment seemed to have initial furcation involvement. This observation, although based on very few cases, supports the findings of Badersten et al.[10] (page 66), Claffey et al.[29] (pages 71-76) and Nordland et al.[72] (pages 78-80).

- In the study by Claffey et al.[29], 22% of furcution sites showed loss of probing attachment over 42 months, as compared with 10% for sites of all surface locations (see page 75). For furcation sites with probing depth ≥ 6 mm and bleeding on probing at 3-month re-evaluation, the corresponding rate of probing attachment loss was 28% (retrospective data analysis).

This suggests that the criterion of probing depth ≥ 6 mm plus bleeding on probing had limited predictive value for probing attachment loss when added to the furcation site location (28% versus 22%).

- The probing measurements at individual sites displayed quite some variability during the 42 months of observation. The graphic presentations of the longitudinal measurements on the preceding pages provide ample evidence of this. It becomes apparent that a comparison of only 2 measurements to determine changes between 2 time points (such as initial and 3 months) may often be flawed. In order to ascertain unequivocal changes it may be necessary to have a series of measurements showing an obvious trend over time. It needs to be pointed out, however, that the case reports included sites with deep probing depths. Reproducibility of probing measurements for deep sites is less than that for shallower sites (see Loos et al.[65], page 44).

- The case reports also illustrate the moderate predictive power of bleeding on probing to disclose loss of probing attachment. Although most of the sites with apparent attachment loss showed bleeding at a majority of examinations during the 42-month interval, there were also sites with stable attachment levels that bled a high number of times. During recording, a positive bleeding score was given for any amount of bleeding visible after probing, including minimal spot-bleeding. This may be a shortcoming, since this type of bleeding may be easily provoked in healthier sites, and perhaps more so in those with deeper probing depths.

- The case reports should be evaluated in view of the following factors:
  - Maintenance care was generally provided twice yearly. The situation at the 3-month re-evaluation may have been altered by subsequent maintenance treatment. If adequate debridement was not accomplished initially but was achieved at a later date, the 3-month re-evaluation status cannot be expected to reflect the outcome of treatment after 42 months. The events for one of the presented cases support this notion (M.B., 21 mesial, page 164).
  - The observation period was limited to 42 months. Given a longer interval, the selected questionable surfaces may have shown more deterioration.

- Only teeth retained throughout the entire 42-month period were included in this chapter. Teeth that were lost due to progressive periodontitis were not included. These teeth constitute the reports in the following chapter.

CHAPTER 6

Case reports – tooth loss

In the preceding chapter of this book, teeth and surfaces with a questionable clinical status at 3-month re-evaluation were presented (pages 129-176). These cases would seem to confirm the limitation of the use of the clinical status at re-evaluation to predict the long-term outcome of treatment, as previously demonstrated from the studies by Badersten et al.[11], Claffey et al.[28,29] and Vanooteghem et al.[94] (pages 112-124). In this chapter, cases with teeth that were lost due to progressive periodontal disease after initial treatment are presented. The clinical status for these teeth prior to treatment, at re-evaluation and during the period leading up to their loss is outlined in order to describe events preceding the tooth loss.

As in the previous chapter, the cases were selected among the 17 patients participating in the study by Claffey et al.[29] (pages 70-77). Five of the 17 patients lost 1-2 teeth due to progressive periodontal disease at some time during the 42 months of observation (total of 6 teeth; see page 76). These teeth were selected for presentation.

The case reports are similar to those in the previous chapter.

CASE A.G.

Age:	61 years
Sex:	Female
Number of remaining teeth:	20 (excluding 1 tooth extracted before treatment)
Tooth lost:	37 (18); after 27 months
Medical history:	None relevant
Medication:	None
Smoker:	No
Dental history:	Regular dental treatment Previous periodontal treatment with unsuccessful outcome

Clinical findings, entire dentition

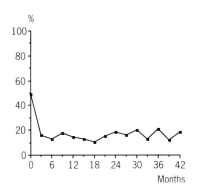

Fig. 6-1. Plaque scores (%)

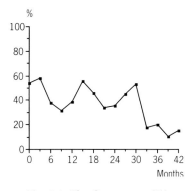

Fig. 6-2. Bleeding scores (%)

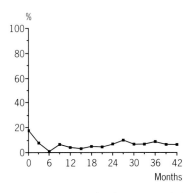

Fig. 6-3. Probing depths ≥ 6 mm (%)

Radiographs, entire dentition

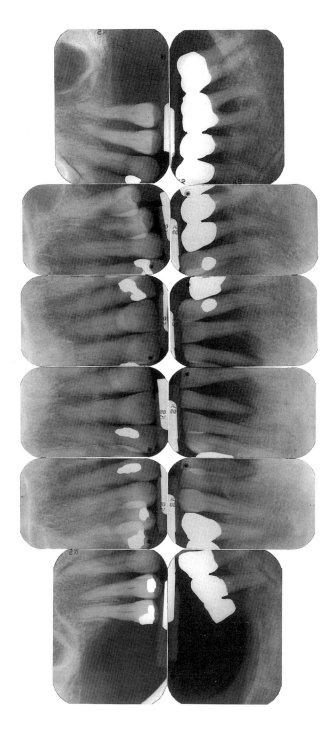

Fig. 6-4

Clinical findings, tooth 37

Table 6-1

Initial

MB	MBM	BF	MBD	**DB***
6.0^{PB}	6.0^{PB}	6.0^{PB}	6.0^{PB}	8.0^{PB}
8.0^{PB}	8.0^{PB}	8.5^{PB}	4.5^{PB}	8.0^{PB}
ML	MLM	LF	**MLD***	DL

3 months

MB	MBM	BF	MBD	**DB***
8.5^{B}	5.0^{B}	6.5^{B}	3.5	7.0
4.5^{B}	7.0	6.0^{B}	4.0^{B}	4.5^{PB}
ML	MLM	LF	**MLD***	DL

27 months

MB	MBM	BF	MBD	**DB***
10.0^{BE}	6.0^{BE}	9.0	3.0	16.0^{B}
9.0^{B}	9.5^{B}	10.0^{B}	10.0^{B}	5.0^{B}
ML	MLM	LF	**MLD***	DL

*The 2 surfaces with greatest attachment loss are indicated in bold (most deteriorating sites).

Radiographs, tooth 37

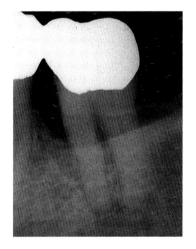
Fig. 6-5. Initial

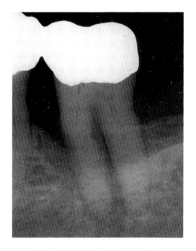
Fig. 6-6. After 27 months

Clinical findings, most deteriorating surfaces, tooth 37

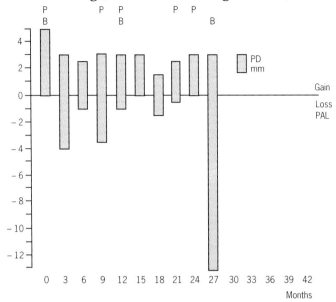

Fig. 6-7. AG, tooth 37, distobuccal

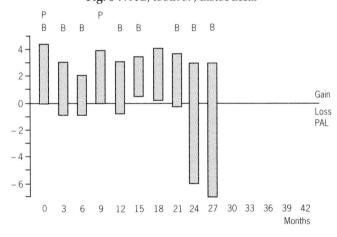

Fig. 6-8. AG, tooth 37, mid-lingual distal root

Comments

- Initially, tooth 37 had the most severe bone loss on the mesial aspect and had furcation involvement buccally and lingually.

- No improvement was observed at 3 months. Patient discomfort and marked deterioration led to the extraction at 27 months. The radiograph from 27 months confirms progression. There is a possibility that the sudden large attachment loss at 24-27 months may have been due to either a periodontal abscess or to the spread of periapical pathology.

CASE C.N.

C.N. was presented in the preceding chapter. See pages 133-136 for general information as well as clinical findings and radiographs from the entire dentition.

Teeth lost: 27 (15); after 39 months
                                            37 (18); after 39 months

Clinical findings, tooth 27

Table 6-2

Initial

	MB	MBM	**BF**	MBD	DB
	7.0^{PB}	-*	8.5^{PB}	-*	7.0^{PB}
	8.5^{PB}		5.0^{P}		7.0^{PB}
	MF		L		DF

3 months

	MB	MBM	**BF**	MBD	DB
	5.0^{B}	-*	5.5^{PB}	-*	5.0^{B}
	5.5^{PB}		5.0^{B}		6.5^{B}
	MF		L		DF

39 months

	MB	MBM	**BF**	MBD	DB
	8.5^{B}	-*	11.0^{PBE}	-*	6.0^{P}
	11.0^{PB}		6.0^{B}		7.0^{PB}
	MF		L		DF

* Findings not available

Radiographs, tooth 27

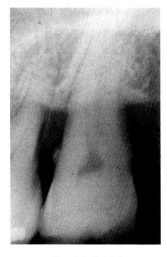

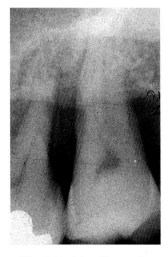

Fig. 6-9. Initial

Fig. 6-10. After 39 months

Clinical findings, most deteriorating surfaces, tooth 27

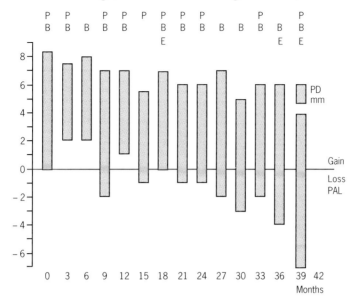

Fig. 6-11. CN, tooth 27, buccal furcation

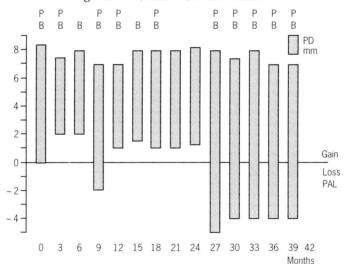

Fig. 6-12. CN, tooth 27, mesial furcation

Comments

- Tooth 27 had marked bone loss initially and furcation involvement of the fused roots from all 3 aspects.

- Improvement was observed at 3 months. However, loss of attachment at 2 of the furcation sites resulted in apical extension of the lesion and pulpal complications. The radiograph from 39 months may reflect the progression.

184

Clinical findings, tooth 37

Table 6-3

Initial

	MB	MBM	**BF**	MBD	DB
	4.5^{PB}	-*	5.0^{PB}	-	5.0^{PB}
	5.0^{PB}	5.0^{P}	6.0^{PB}	4.5^{PB}	5.0^{PB}
	ML	MLM	**LF**	MLD	DL

3 months

	MB	MBM	**BF**	MBD	DB
	3.0^{B}	-	4.5	-	5.5^{P}
	4.5^{PB}	5.0^{PB}	6.0^{PB}	4.0^{B}	4.5^{PB}
	ML	MLM	**LF**	MLD	DL

39 months

	MB	MBM	**BF**	MBD	DB
	4.5^{B}	-	12.0^{B}	-	5.0^{B}
	7.0^{B}	6.0^{B}	14.0^{B}	10.0^{B}	5.0^{B}
	ML	MLM	**LF**	MLD	DL

* Findings not available

Radiographs, tooth 37

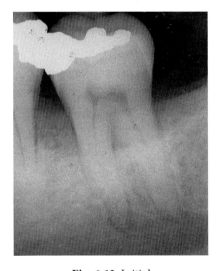

Fig. 6-13. Initial

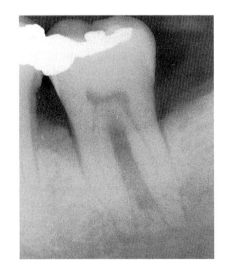

Fig. 6-14. After 39 months

Clinical findings, most deteriorating surfaces, tooth 37

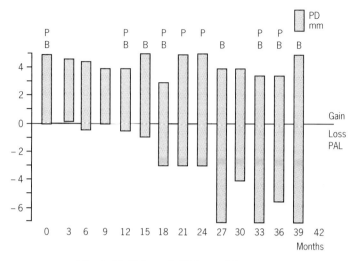

Fig. 6-15. CN, tooth 37, buccal furcation

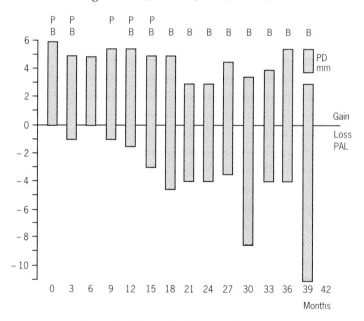

Fig. 6-16. CN, tooth 37, lingual furcation

Comments

- Initially, tooth 37 had some bone loss and furcation involvement from the lingual aspect.

- Gradual deterioration in the furcation areas led to apical extension of the lesion and pulpal complications. The radiograph at 39 months confirms the progression.

CASE J.O.

J.O. was presented in the preceding chapter. See pages 145-148 for general information as well as clinical findings and radiographs from the entire dentition.

Tooth lost: 16 (3); after 21 months

Clinical findings, tooth 16

Table 6-4

Initial

	DB	MBD	BF	**MBM**	MB
	11.0^{PBE}	8.0^{PB}	7.0^{PB}	7.5^{B}	11.0^{B}
	7.5^{PB}		4.0^{PB}		9.0^{PB}
	DF		L		**MF**

3 months

	DB	MBD	BF	**MBM**	MB
	8.0^{B}	6.5	6.0^{B}	8.5	10.0^{B}
	4.5		3.5		11.0
	DF		L		**MF**

21 months

	DB	MBD	BF	**MBM**	MB
	8.0^{B}	6.5^{B}	6.0^{B}	10.5^{B}	11.5^{B}
	6.0^{B}		3.5^{P}		11.0^{B}
	DF		L		**MF**

Radiograph, tooth 16

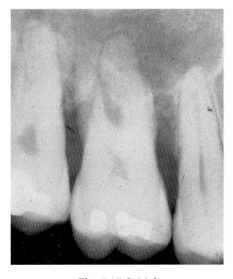

Fig. 6-17. Initial

Clinical findings, most deteriorating surfaces, tooth 16

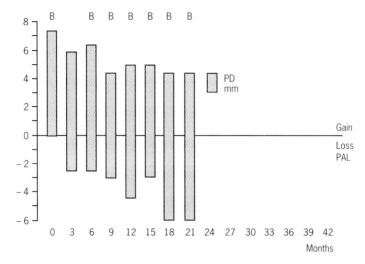

Fig. 6-18. JO, tooth 16, mid-buccal mesial root

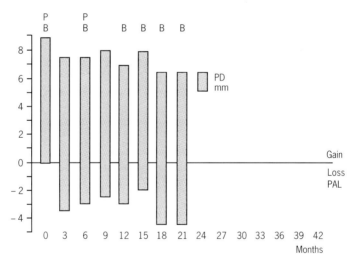

Fig. 6-19. JO, tooth 16, mesial furcation

Comments

- Initially, tooth 16 had advanced bone loss and furcation involvement from all 3 aspects.

- Gradual deterioration around the mesial root led to apical extension of the lesion and patient discomfort.

CASE J.S.

J.S. was presented in the preceding chapter. See pages 149-152 for general information as well as clinical findings and radiographs from the entire dentition.

Tooth lost: 27 (15); after 27 months

Clinical findings, tooth 27

Table 6-5

Initial

MB	MBM	BF	MBD	**DB**
7.0^{PB}	3.0^{PB}	4.5^{PB}	4.0^{PB}	5.0^{P}
10.0^{PB}		6.0^{PB}		8.0^{PB}
MF		L		**DF**

3 months

MB	MBM	BF	MBD	**DB**
2.0^{B}	2.0	3.0^{PB}	3.0	8.5
6.5^{B}		3.0		8.5^{B}
MF		L		**DF**

27 months

MB	MBM	BF	MBD	**DB**
2.0	2.0	3.0^{PB}	2.0	10.5^{B}
10.0^{B}		3.0^{B}		8.0^{B}
MF		L		**DF**

Radiographs, tooth 27

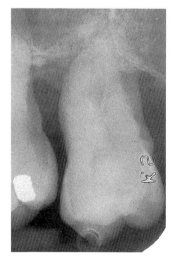

Fig. 6-20. Initial

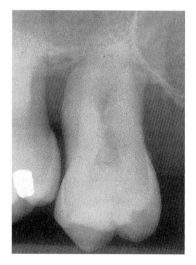

Fig. 6-21. After 24 months

Clinical findings, most deteriorating surfaces, tooth 27

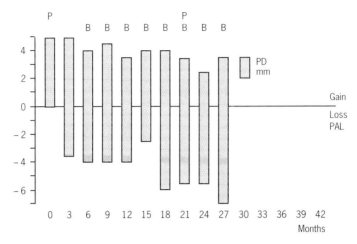

Fig. 6-22. JS, tooth 27, distobuccal

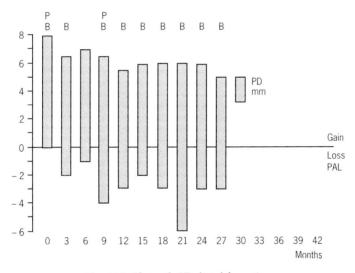

Fig. 6-23. JS, tooth 27, distal furcation

Comments

- Initially, tooth 27 had advanced bone loss and furcation involvement from all 3 aspects.

- Gradual deterioration resulted in apical extension of the periodontal lesions and patient discomfort.

- The radiograph at 24 months would also seem to indicate progression.

CASE L.V.

Age:	34 years
Sex:	Male
Number of remaining teeth:	18
Tooth lost:	25 (13); after 36 months
Medical history:	None relevant
Medication:	No
Smoker:	No
Dental history:	Sporadic dental treatment
	No previous periodontal treatment

Clinical findings, entire dentition

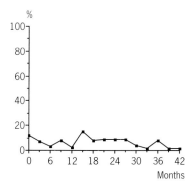

Fig. 6-24. Plaque scores (%)

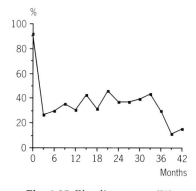

Fig. 6-25. Bleeding scores (%)

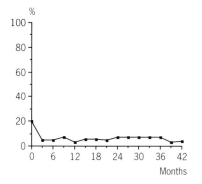

Fig. 6-26. Probing depths ≥ 6 mm (%)

Radiographs, entire dentition

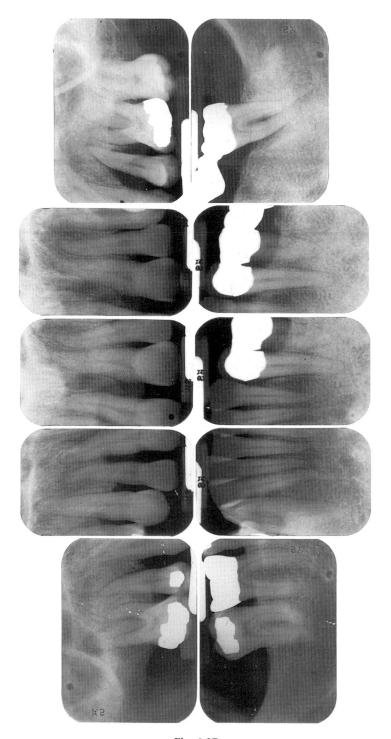

Fig. 6-27

Clinical findings, tooth 25

Table 6-6

Initial

MB	B	DB
8.0^B	4.0^B	7.0^B
8.5^B	5.0^B	8.0^B
ML	**L**	DL

3 months

MB	B	DB
8.5^{PB}	3.5^B	5.5
7.0^B	4.5^B	5.0^B
ML	**L**	DL

36 months

MB	B	DB
7.5	3.0	6.0
7.0^B	8.0	5.0^B
ML	**L**	DL

Radiographs, tooth 25

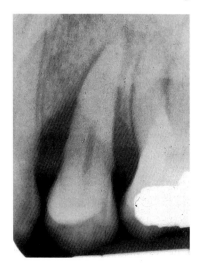
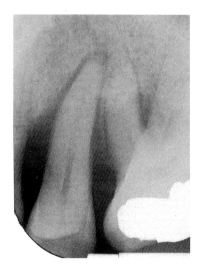

Fig. 6-28. Initial   **Fig. 6-29**. After 27 months

Clinical findings, most deteriorating surfaces, tooth 25

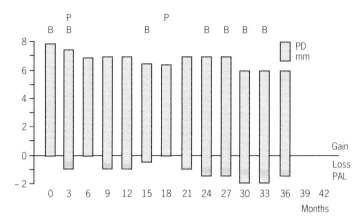

Fig. 6-30. LV, tooth 25, mesiobuccal

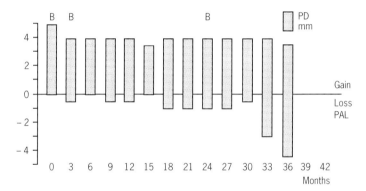

Fig. 6-31. LV, tooth 25, lingual

Comments

- Tooth 25 showed initial mobility, advanced bone loss and mesial and distal intraosseous defects.

- At 33 months the tooth started to cause discomfort to the patient. Deterioration took place primarily on the lingual aspect and resulted in apical extension of the lesion.

- The radiograph at 27 months did not reveal any progression at that time.

GENERAL COMMENTS

- Five of 6 teeth that were lost due to progressive periodontitis among the 17 treated patients had furcation involvement initially. This, again, reinforces the compromised prognosis for some of the teeth with such involvement.

- All teeth that were lost had deep, bleeding sites at 3-month re-evaluation. Along with the loss of attachment, the probing depths deepened and the number of bleeding sites around the teeth tended to increase. This material cannot be used to assess the predictive power of residual probing depths and bleeding, as the teeth were selected on the basis of their demise. Nevertheless, it does demonstrate that deep pockets and bleeding are part of the disease process. The apparent difficulty at re-evaluation is undoubtedly the separation of the lesions that might continue to progress from those that will remain stable.

- The number and type of teeth lost during the first couple of years after periodontal therapy is obviously a function of the criteria used for extraction prior to therapy. Therapists may claim that some of the teeth presented above had a hopeless prognosis and should have been removed initially. However, the subjects participated in a study with a protocol that called for treatment of all periodontally involved teeth unless they had lesions extending to the root apex.

CHAPTER 7

Considerations for clinical practice

Our present methods for clinical evaluation of marginal periodontal tissues include the use of bleeding, suppuration and probing depth. There is little doubt that these methods provide useful guidelines for evaluation of the overall periodontal status of dentitions.

On an individual site basis, these methods have limitations in the identification of locations prone to disease progression. So far, there is no reliable clinical, microbiological or other method to predict or identify sites with disease activity (ongoing loss of attachment). Therefore, active lesions have to be distinguished from arrested lesions without clear guidelines.

A treatment resulting in a plaque-free mouth with nonbleeding, shallow probing depths throughout the dentition will reduce the risk of residual, active lesions. Such a result, although desirable, is not realistic for many patients. Therefore, the clinician is faced with the delicate task of evaluating sites with various grades of involvement using current clinical methods of examination.

Time for re-evaluation

Traditionally, re-evaluation is performed a few months after initial periodontal treatment. The results of clinical research suggest that 3 months posttreatment is a suitable interval for primary re-evaluation. Most of the clinical healing has occurred at this time, even in areas with deep lesions initially.

Continuous progression of periodontal disease after initial treatment is a slow process in the vast majority of chronic periodontitis patients. This seems to be valid even for the patients thought to be most susceptible because of advanced periodontal destruction at the time of diagnosis. From this viewpoint, there is limited need to initiate supplementary surgical therapy at an early time. Repeated measurements would seem to increase the diagnostic validity of our clinical scores, thereby leading to a lesser likelihood of overtreatment. When practical circumstances allow, repeated evaluations over a couple of years may be the procedure of choice in situations where the need for re-treatment is less than obvious.

For monitoring purposes in susceptible individuals, recordings of probing depths at yearly intervals and identification of sites with increase in probing depth would seem to constitute a feasible approach. Sites identified in this way should be considered for re-treatment, particularly if they bleed easily on probing.

Plaque scores

The fact that the presence of supragingival plaque so far has been found to have little or no association with disease progression does not lessen the importance of good plaque control for our patients. Absence of supragingival plaque would still seem to be the best guarantee against probing attachment loss due to inflammatory periodontal disease.

Bleeding scores

The limited to moderate predictive value of bleeding on probing for disease activity, as observed from the studies reviewed, may be related to the fact that a positive bleeding score has been given for any amount of bleeding visible after probing, including minimal spot-bleeding. It is possible that improved predictive power would have been found if only more obvious amounts of bleeding provoked with light probing pressure had been registered. The clinician may primarily suspect ongoing disease activity if the tissues bleed easily and markedly. However, it is still open to question whether bleeding on probing as the only sign of residual disease justifies immediate re-treatment.

Suppuration on probing

The determination of the predictive value of suppuration on probing has been hampered by its infrequent occurrence after initial therapy. From a biological point of view, it seems reasonable to assume that subgingival accumulation of pus, to the extent that it can be observed clinically, is a sign of potential or ongoing disease activity. In spite of the finding of a moderate predictive power, the occurrence of either suppuration on probing or spontaneous suppuration would seem to warrant re-treatment.

Probe penetration

Prior to treatment, a thin probe tip (diameter 0.35-0.40 mm) combined with a low to moderate probing force (0.25-0.50 N) generally penetrates to the apical termination of the junctional epithelium or slightly beyond into the connective tissue. As a result of initial treatment, particularly for sites with deep probing depth, the probe tip will commonly stop 1-2 mm coronal to the base of the junctional epithelium. This gain in probing attachment is the result of improved gingival health and improved tissue tonus offering more resistance to probe penetration. The clinician needs to keep this histological background in mind during evaluation and monitoring of patients. The observation of a larger probing depth after treatment than before treatment is most likely a reflection of loss of connective tissue attachment (unless there has been a significant swelling of the gingiva – a rare observation). A larger probing depth recorded at a later posttreatment time compared with a previous posttreatment time may not be related to loss of connective tissue attachment. Instead, it may be due to a reduction in tissue tonus allowing the probe to penetrate more deeply along the junctional epithelium.

Probing force

Probing forces ranging from 0.25 N to 0.75 N have most often been used in the studies reviewed. Although standardization of the probing force is a requirement for clinical research, it may not be practical for clinical practice. The clinician will often experience a need to use greater force at some locations in the dentition due to anatomical and other reasons. In addition, the clinician may adjust the probing force to the level of pain tolerance of the individual patient. One should be aware, however, that variation of the probing force will result in variation of recorded probing depth.

Reproducibility of probing

Variations in the location of the probe at the examination sites together with differences in probe angulation are probably the most common causes of lack of reproducibility of probing recordings. These variations may occur more commonly if the connective tissue attachment at the site has an oblique or irregular course. For clinical purposes, differences between examinations of 1 mm only should be considered as due to probing errors. Differences of 2 mm, less likely to reflect probing error, may be more clinically significant. It may be practical to use this difference to indicate change.

Probing depth

In the past, sites with residual probing depths of a given magnitude (such as ≥ 5 mm or ≥ 6 mm) have often been considered to be a result of unsuccessful treatment and should therefore be re-treated with subgingival debridement or subjected to surgical treatment. Findings from more recent research, including those reviewed in this book, have indicated that such an approach may be questionable. Although a deeper probing depth might reflect the history of previous disease, it may not be a sign of ongoing disease activity. The residual probing depth at a given site should be evaluated relative to the depth prior to treatment. A reduction in depth would seem to be an indication of improvement, even if the posttreatment depth is relatively great. Conversely, an increase in depth indicates deterioration, even if the posttreatment depth is comparatively shallow.

Routines for clinical practice should be designed to facilitate the detection of probing depth changes between successive recordings. Due to the magnitude of change needed to overcome probing reproducibility error and due to the slow progression of the disease, a prolonged period of monitoring may be necessary to detect meaningful changes.

Radiographic evaluation

The radiographic image of the marginal periodontal bone may vary with the X-ray projection used and probably also with other factors related to exposure and development of the films. Lack of standardization may be one of the reasons why the perceived presence or absence of a crestal lamina dura has been found to be unrelated to the inflammatory status of the gingiva. One also encounters difficulties in the exact identification of the coronal bone margin.

Due to these difficulties, conventional radiographs cannot be used to detect minor changes in periodontal bone height following initial periodontal treatment. Therefore, it would seem that routine radiographs taken at re-evaluation for the purpose of comparison to radiographs obtained prior to treatment are of little value. Radiographic comparisons are primarily useful as a supplementary diagnostic tool when greater changes in the marginal bone are suspected at later maintenance intervals.

Subgingival calculus detection

Although large amounts of subgingival calculus prior to treatment may be detected by probing, smaller amounts remaining after subgingival debridement performed by a trained clinician will probably not be disclosed. This would seem to hold true also for radiographic detection of calculus on approximal surfaces. Once a clinician has acquired the necessary clinical skill, the effectiveness of subgingival debridement seems to be best evaluated from assessment of the inflammatory status of the gingiva.

Probing attachment loss

In each of the studies demonstrating the effect of initial periodontal treatment, a given proportion of sites continued to lose probing attachment. As pointed out above, we do not yet have a reliable method of determining disease activity. As a consequence, we cannot distinguish lesions with active disease from quiescent lesions or from lesions with ongoing attachment loss due to reasons other than disease. Interpretation of probing attachment level data for the purpose of attempting to evaluate the risk to patients of disease progression is therefore difficult.

Probing attachment level measurements are not usually recorded in clinical practice due to the cumbersome nature of the measurements. Assuming that such recordings had been obtained to monitor the effect of treatment, one would have been faced with the problem of deciding which sites with probing attachment loss had deteriorated due to inflammatory periodontal disease and which showed probing attachment loss due to other reasons. In such a situation, requirements of bleeding on probing and increase in probing depth in addition to probing attachment loss would seem to enhance the likelihood of identification of sites with true periodontal disease.

Susceptibility to periodontal disease

As would be expected, research has demonstrated that previous exposure to periodontal disease is an indication of the risk of additional deterioration. Currently, there are no other methods to judge patient susceptibility to the reoccurrence of disease (apart from some systemic diseases affecting the immune system). For clinical practice, this means that the evaluation and monitoring of treatment should be related to the rate of previous disease progression, taking the amount of periodontal destruction and the age of the patient into consideration. Recall intervals should be short and completeness of records without compromise for a patient who has incurred severely advanced disease before the age of 30 years. A patient at the age of 60 years who has never been treated for periodontal disease and with an abundance of plaque and calculus would be expected to show a good response to treatment and to require more limited recall and maintenance.

Facing the challenge

As should be obvious from the content of this book, the lack of guidelines for periodontal evaluation creates a situation in which overtreatment is one end of the scale and "supervised neglect" the other. Despite this lack of knowledge, the clinician is expected to make decisions that should consider both the needs of the individual patient and the current state of the art. The latter includes the base of knowledge acquired from research as well as the current and accepted mode of clinical practice. Since our understanding is continuously widening, the clinician is obligated to be updated at all times in order to provide adequate service to the patients.

CHAPTER 8

References

1. Albandar JM, Rise J, Gjermo P, Johansen JR. Radiographic quantification of alveolar bone level changes. A 2-year longitudinal study in man. J Clin Periodontol 1986; 13: 195-200.

2. Axelsson P, Lindhe J. Effect of controlled oral hygiene procedures on caries and periodontal disease in adults. Results after 6 years. J Clin Periodontol 1981; 8: 239-48.

3. Badersten A. Effect of nonsurgical periodontal therapy. Thesis. Lund, Sweden: University of Lund, 1984.

4. Badersten A, Nilvéus R, Egelberg J. Effect of nonsurgical periodontal therapy. II. Severely advanced periodontitis. J Clin Periodontol 1984; 11: 63-76.

5. Badersten A, Nilvéus R, Egelberg J. Effect of nonsurgical periodontal therapy. III. Single versus repeated instrumentation. J Clin Periodontol 1984; 11: 114-24.

6. Badersten A, Nilvéus R, Egelberg J. Reproducibility of probing attachment level measurements. J Clin Periodontol 1984; 11: 475-85.

7. Badersten A, Nilvéus R, Egelberg J. Effect of nonsurgical periodontal therapy. IV. Operator variability. J Clin Periodontol 1985; 12: 190-200.

8. Badersten A, Nilvéus R, Egelberg J. Effect of nonsurgical periodontal therapy. VI. Localization of sites with probing attachment loss. J Clin Periodontol 1985; 12: 351-9.

9. Badersten A, Nilvéus R, Egelberg J. Effect of nonsurgical periodontal therapy. VII. Bleeding, suppuration and probing depth in sites with probing attachment loss. J Clin Periodontol 1985; 12: 432-40.

10. Badersten A, Nilvéus R, Egelberg J. Effect of nonsurgical periodontal therapy. VIII. Probing attachment changes related to clinical characteristics. J Clin Periodontol 1987; 14: 425-32.

11. Badersten A, Nilvéus R, Egelberg J. Scores of plaque, bleeding, suppuration and probing depth to predict probing attachment loss. 5 years of observation following nonsurgical periodontal therapy. J Clin Periodontol 1990; 17: 102-7.

12. Badersten A, Nilvéus R, Egelberg J. Effect of nonsurgical periodontal therapy. Radiographic alterations. Unpublished.

13. Best AM, Burmeister JA, Gunsolley JC, Brooks CN, Schenkein HA. Reliability of attachment loss measurements in a longitudinal clinical trial. J Clin Periodontol 1990; 17: 564-9.

14. Biller IR, Kerber PE. Reliability of scaling error detection. J Dent Educ 1980; 44: 206-10.

15. Bolin A, Lavstedt S, Henrikson CO. Proximal alveolar bone loss in a longitudinal radiographic investigation. III. Some predictors with a possible influence on the progression in an unselected material. Acta Odontol Scand 1986; 44: 257-62.

16. Brayer WK, Mellonig JT, Dunlop RM, Marinak KW, Carson RE. Scaling and root planing effectiveness: the effect of root surface access and operator experience. J Periodontol 1989; 60: 67-72.

17. Buchanan SA, Robertson PA. Calculus removal by scaling/root planing with and without surgical access. J Periodontol 1987; 58: 159-63.

18. Buckley LA, Crowley MJ. A longitudinal study of untreated periodontal dis-

ease. J Clin Periodontol 1984; 11: 523-30.

19. Caffesse RG, Sweeney PL, Smith BA. Scaling and root planing with and without periodontal flap surgery. J Clin Periodontol 1986; 13: 205-10.

20. Caton J, Greenstein G, Polson AM. Depth of periodontal probe penetration related to clinical and histologic signs of gingival inflammation. J Periodontol 1981; 52: 626-9.

21. Caton J, Proye M, Polson AM. Maintenance of healed periodontal pockets after a single episode of root planing. J Periodontol 1982; 53: 420-4.

22. Cercek JF, Kiger RD, Garrett S, Egelberg J. Relative effects of plaque control and instrumentation on the clinical parameters of periodontal disease. J Clin Periodontol 1983; 10: 46-56.

23. Chamberlain ADH, Renvert S, Garrett S, Nilvéus R, Egelberg J. Significance of probing force for evaluation of healing following periodontal therapy. J Clin Periodontol 1985; 12: 306-11.

24. Chaves ES, Caffesse RG, Morrison EC, Stults DL. Diagnostic discrimination of bleeding on probing during maintenance periodontal therapy. Am J Dent 1990; 3: 167-70.

25. Claffey N. Decision making in periodontal therapy. The re-evaluation. J Clin Periodontol 1991; 18: 384-9.

26. Claffey N, Egelberg J. Clinical characteristics of periodontal sites with probing attachment loss following initial periodontal treatment. J Clin Periodontol (in press).

27. Claffey N, Loos B, Gantes B, Martin M, Heins P, Egelberg J. The relative effects of therapy and periodontal disease on loss of probing attachment after root debridement. J Clin Periodontol 1988; 15: 163-9.

28. Claffey N, Loos B, Gantes B, Martin M, Egelberg J. Probing depth at re-evaluation following initial periodontal therapy to indicate the initial response to treatment. J Clin Periodontol 1989; 16: 229-33.

29. Claffey N, Nylund K, Kiger R, Garrett S, Egelberg J. Diagnostic predictability of scores of plaque, bleeding, suppuration and probing depth for probing attachment loss. 3.5 years of observation following initial periodontal therapy. J Clin Periodontol 1990; 17: 108-14.

30. Davenport RH, Simpson DM, Hassell TM. Histometric comparison of active and inactive lesions of advanced periodontitis. J Periodontol 1982; 53: 285-95.

31. Dubrez B, Graf JM, Vaugnat P, Cimasoni G. Increase of interproximal bone density after subgingival instrumentation: a quantitative radiographic study. J Periodontol 1990; 61: 725-31.

32. Egelberg J. The impact of regression towards the mean on probing changes in studies on the effect of periodontal therapy. J Clin Periodontol 1989; 16: 120-3.

33. Egelberg J. Periodontics - the scientific way. Copenhagen: Munksgaard, 1992: 60-98.

34. Fleischer HC, Mellonig JT, Brayer WK, Gray JL, Barnett JD. Scaling and root planing efficacy in multirooted teeth. J Periodontol 1989; 60: 402-9.

35. Fowler C, Garrett S, Crigger M, Egelberg J. Histologic probe position in treated and untreated human periodontal tissues. J Clin Periodontol 1982; 9: 373-85.

36. Freed HK, Gapper RJ, Kalkwarf KL. Evaluation of periodontal probing forces. J Periodontol 1983; 54: 488-92.

37. Garnick JJ, Spray JR, Vernino DM, Klawitter JJ. Demonstration of periodontal probes in human periodontal pockets. J Periodontol 1980; 51: 563-70.

38. Glavind L, Löe H. Errors in the clinical assessment of periodontal destruction. J Periodont Res 1967; 2: 180-4.

39. Goodson JM, Tanner ACR, Haffajee AD, Sornberger GC, Socransky SS. Patterns of progression and regression of advanced destructive periodontal disease. J Clin Periodontol 1982; 9: 472-81.

40. Grbic JT, Lamster IB. Risk indicators for future clinical attachment loss in adult periodontitis. Tooth and site variables. J Periodontol 1992; 63: 262-9.

41. Grbic JT, Lamster IB, Celenti RS, Fine JB. Risk indicators for future clinical attachment loss in adult periodontitis. Patient variables. J Periodontol 1991; 62: 322-9.

42. Greenstein G, Polson A, Iker H, Meitner S. Associations between crestal lamina dura and periodontal status. J Periodontol 1981; 52: 362-6.

43. Greenstein G, Caton J, Polson A. Histologic characteristics associated with bleeding after probing and visual signs of inflammation. J Periodontol 1981; 52: 420-5.

44. Haffajee AD, Socransky SS, Goodson JM. Comparison of different data analyses for detecting changes in attachment level. J Clin Periodontol 1983; 10: 298-310.

45. Haffajee AD, Socransky SS, Lindhe J, Okamoto H, Yoneyama T. Clinical risk indicators for periodontal attachment loss. J Clin Periodontol 1991; 18: 117-25.

46. Halazonetis TD, Haffajee AD, Socransky SS. Relationship of clinical parameters to attachment loss in subsets of subjects with destructive periodontal diseases. J Clin Periodontol 1989; 16: 563-8.

47. Harper DS, Robinson PJ. Correlation of histometric, microbial, and clinical indicators of periodontal disease status before and after root planing. J Clin Periodontol 1987; 14: 190-6.

48. Hassell TM, Germann MA, Saxer UP. Periodontal probing: interinvestigator discrepancies and correlations between probing force and recorded depth. Helv Odontol Acta 1973; 17: 38-42.

49. Heft MW, Perelmuter SH, Cooper BY, Magnusson I, Clark WB. Relationship between gingival inflammation and painfulness of periodontal probing. J Clin Periodontol 1991; 18: 213-15.

50. Isidor F, Karring T, Attström R. Reproducibility of pocket depth and attachment level measurements when using a flexible splint. J Clin Periodontol 1984; 11: 662-8.

51. Isidor F, Attström R, Karring T. Regeneration of alveolar bone following surgical and non-surgical periodontal treatment. J Clin Periodontol 1985; 12: 687-96.

52. Janssen PTM, Faber JAJ, van Palenstein Helderman WH. Reproducibility of bleeding tendency measurements and the reproducibility of mouth bleeding scores for the individual patient. J Periodont Res 1986; 21: 653-9.

53. Janssen PTM, Faber JAJ, van Palenstein Helderman WH. Non-Gaussian distribution of differences between duplicate probing depth measurements. J Clin Periodontol 1987; 14: 345-9.

54. Janssen PTM, Faber JAJ, van Palenstein Helderman WH. Effect of probing depth and bleeding tendency on the reproducibility of probing depth measurements. J Clin Periodontol 1988; 15: 565-8.

55. Janssen PTM, Drayer A, Faber JAJ, van Palenstein Helderman WH. Accuracy of repeated single versus average of repeated duplicates of probing depth measurements. J Clin Periodontol 1988; 15: 569-74.

56. Jenkins WMM, MacFarlane TW, Gilmour WH. Longitudinal study of untreated periodontitis. I. Clinical findings. J Clin Periodontol 1988; 15: 324-30.

57. Karayiannis A, Lang NP, Joss A, Nyman S. Bleeding on probing as it re-

lates to probing pressure and gingival health in patients with a reduced but healthy periodontium. J Clin Periodontol 1992; 19: 471-5.

58. Lang NP, Joss A, Orsanic T, Gusberti FA, Siegrist BE. Bleeding on probing. A predictor for the progression of periodontal disease? J Clin Periodontol 1986; 13: 590-6.

59. Lang NP, Adler R, Joss A, Nyman S. Absence of bleeding on probing. An indicator of periodontal stability. J Clin Periodontol 1990; 17: 714-21.

60. Lang NP, Nyman S, Senn C, Joss A. Bleeding on probing as is relates to probing pressure and gingival health. J Clin Periodontol 1991; 18: 257-61.

61. Lindhe J, Haffajee AD, Socransky SS. Progression of periodontal disease in adult subjects in the absence of periodontal therapy. J Clin Periodontol 1983; 10: 433-42.

62. Lindhe J, Okamoto H, Yoneyama T, Haffajee A, Socransky SS. Periodontal loser sites in untreated adult subjects. J Clin Periodontol 1989; 16: 662-70.

63. Lindhe J, Okamoto H, Yoneyama T, Haffajee A, Socransky SS. Longitudinal changes in periodontal disease in untreated subjects. J Clin Periodontol 1989; 16: 671-8.

64. Löe H, Anerud A, Boysen H, Morrison E. Natural history of periodontal disease in man. J Clin Periodontol 1986; 13: 431-40.

65. Loos B, Kiger R, Egelberg J. An evaluation of basic periodontal therapy using sonic and ultrasonic scalers. J Clin Periodontol 1987; 14: 29-33.

66. Loos B, Claffey N, Egelberg J. Clinical and microbial effects of root debridement in periodontal furcation pockets. J Clin Periodontol 1988; 15: 453-63.

67. Loos B, Nylund K, Claffey N, Egelberg J. Clinical effects of root debridement in molar and non-molar teeth. A 2-year follow-up. J Clin Periodontol 1989; 16: 498-504.

68. Magnusson I, Fuller WW, Heins PJ, Rau CF, Gibbs CH, Clark WB. Correlation between electronic and visual readings of pocket depths with a newly developed constant force probe. J Clin Periodontol 1988; 15: 180-4.

69. Marks RG, Low SB, Taylor M, Baggs R, Magnusson I, Clark WB. Reproducibility of attachment level measurements with two models of the Florida probe. J Clin Periodontol 1991; 18: 780-4.

70. Matia JI, Bissada NF, Maybury JE, Riccetti P. Efficiency of scaling of the molar furcation area with and without surgical access. Int J Periodont Restorative Dent 1986; 6: 25-35.

71. Moriarty JD, Hutchens LH, Scheitler LE. Histological evaluation of periodontal probe penetration in untreated facial molar furcations. J Clin Periodontol 1989; 16: 21-6.

72. Nordland P, Garrett S, Kiger R, Vanooteghem R, Hutchens LH, Egelberg J. The effect of plaque control and root debridement in molar teeth. J Clin Periodontol 1987; 14: 231-6.

73. Nylund K, Egelberg J. Antimicrobial irrigation of periodontal furcation lesions to supplement oral hygiene instruction and root debridement. J Clin Periodontol 1990; 17: 90-5.

74. Okano T, Mera T, Ohki M, Ishikawa I, Yamada N. Digital subtraction of radiographs in evaluating alveolar bone changes after initial periodontal therapy. Oral Surg Oral Med Oral Pathol 1990; 69: 258-62.

75. Osborn JB, Stoltenberg JL, Huso BA, Aeppli DM, Pihlstrom BL. Comparison of measurement variability in subjects with moderate periodontitis using a conventional and constant force periodontal probe. J Periodontol 1992; 63: 283-9.

76. Papapanou PN, Wennström JL. The angular bone defect as indicator of further alveolar bone loss. J Clin Periodontol 1991; 18: 317-22.

77. Papapanou PN, Wennström JL, Gröndahl KA. 10-year retrospective study of periodontal disease progression. J Clin Periodontol 1989; 16: 403-11.

78. Passo SA, Reinhardt RA, DuBois LM, Cohen DM. Histological characteristics associated with suppurating periodontal pockets. J Periodontol 1988; 59: 731-40.

79. Pippin DJ, Feil P. Interrater agreement on subgingival calculus detection following scaling. J Dent Educ 1992; 56: 322-6.

80. Polson AM, Caton JG, Yeaple RN, Zander HA. Histologic determination of probe tip penetration into gingival sulcus of humans using an electronic pressure-sensitive probe. J Clin Periodontol 1980; 7: 479-88.

81. Proye M, Caton J, Polson A. Initial healing of periodontal pockets after a single episode of root planing monitored by controlled probing forces. J Periodontol 1982; 53: 296-301.

82. Rabbani GM, Ash MM, Caffesse RG. The effectiveness of subgingival scaling and root planing in calculus removal. J Periodontol 1981; 52: 119-23.

83. Robinson PJ, Vitek RM. The relationship between gingival inflammation and resistance to probe penetration. J Periodont Res 1979; 14: 239-43.

84. Schmidt EF, Webber RL, Ruttimann UE, Loesche WJ. Effect of periodontal therapy on alveolar bone as measured by subtraction radiography. J Periodontol 1988; 59: 633-8.

85. Sherman PR, Hutchens LH, Jewson LG, Moriarty JM, Greco GW, McFall WT. The effectiveness of subgingival scaling and root planing. I. Clinical detection of residual calculus. J Periodontol 1990; 61: 3-8.

86. Sherman PR, Hutchens LH, Jewson LG. The effectiveness of subgingival scaling and root planing. II. Clinical response related to residual calculus. J Periodontol 1990; 61: 9-15.

87. Simons P, Watts T. Validity of a hinged constant force probe and a similar, immobilized probe in untreated periodontal disease. J Clin Periodontol 1987; 14: 581-7.

88. Spray JR, Garnick JJ, Doles LR, Klawitter JJ. Microscopic demonstration of the position of periodontal probes. J Periodontol 1978; 49: 148-52.

89. van der Velden U. Probing force and the relationship of the probe tip to the periodontal tissues. J Clin Periodontol 1979; 6: 106-14.

90. van der Velden U. Influence of periodontal health on probing depth and bleeding tendency. J Clin Periodontol 1980; 7: 129-39.

91. van der Velden U. Location of probe tip in bleeding and non-bleeding pockets with minimal gingival inflammation. J Clin Periodontol 1982; 9: 421-7.

92. van der Velden U, de Vries JH. The influence of probing force on the reproducibility of pocket depth measurements. J Clin Periodontol 1980; 7: 414-20.

93. Vanooteghem R, Hutchens LH, Garrett S, Kiger R, Egelberg J. Bleeding on probing and probing depth as indicators of the response to plaque control and root debridement. J Clin Periodontol 1987; 14: 226-30.

94. Vanooteghem R, Hutchens LH, Bowers G, Kramer G, Schallhorn R, Kiger R, Crigger M, Egelberg J. Subjective criteria and probing attachment loss to evaluate the effects of plaque control and root debridement. J Clin Periodontol 1990; 17: 580-7.

95. Watts T. Constant force probing with and without a stent in untreated periodontal disease: the clinical reproducibility problem and possible sources of error. J Clin Periodontol 1987; 14: 407-11.

CHAPTER 9

Index

The page references for each of the 3 chapters refer to pages where data on indicated items can be found.

Chapter 2. Methods of evaluation

Chapter 3. Effect of initial periodontal treatment

Chapter 4. Prediction and evaluation of deterioration